Dedicated to Albrecht,
who is no longer with us

Springer

Milan
Berlin
Heidelberg
New York
Hong Kong
London
Paris
Tokyo

L. Solbiati · A. Martegani · E. Leen · J.M. Correas
P.N. Burns · D. Becker

Contrast-Enhanced Ultrasound of Liver Diseases

With contributions by

L. Aiani · A. Bauer · A. Bellobuono · C. Borghi · L. Cova
O. Hélénon · V. Kirn · V. Osti · M. Tonolini

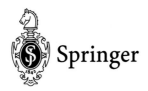

Springer

Dr. Luigi Solbiati
Chairman, Dept. of Radiology
General Hospital
Piazzale Solaro 3
21052 Busto Arsizio (VA), Italy

Dr. Alberto Martegani
Servizio di Radiologia
Ospedale Valduce
Via Dante 11
I-22100 Como, Italy

Dr. Edward Leen
Consultant Radiologist/Senior Lecturer
University of Glasgow
Dept. of Radiology
Royal Infirmary
Alexandra Parade
Glasgow G31 2ER, UK

Dr. Jean Michel Correas
Service de Radiologie Adulte
Hôpital Necker Enfants Malades
149 rue de Sèvres
75743 Paris Cédex 15, France

Dr. Peter N. Burns
Depts. of Medical Biophysics and
Radiology
University of Toronto
Sunnybrook and Women's Health
Sciences Centre
Toronto, Canada

Dr. Dirk Becker
Chairman, Dept. of Medicine
Gastroenterology, Intensive Care
Medicine
Eckernförde Community Hospital
Schleswiger Str. 114 - 116
D-24340 Eckernförde, Germany

Contributors

L. Aiani • A. Bauer[†] • A. Bellobuono • C. Borghi • L. Cova
O. Hélénon • V. Kirn • V. Osti • M. Tonolini

Springer-Verlag Italia
a member of BertelsmannSpringer Science+Business Media GmbH

http://www.springer.de

© Springer-Verlag Italia, Milano 2003

ISBN 88-470-0207-9

Library of Congress Cataloging-in-Publication Data: applied for

Typesetting: Compostudio, Cernusco sul Naviglio (Milano)
Printing and binding: Staroffset, Cernusco sul Naviglio (Milano)
Cover design: Simona Colombo (Milano)

Printed in Italy

SPIN: 10904398

Preface

In the last few years, the development of sonographic contrast agents – or "microbubbles" – has stimulated increasingly intensive studies on the relationships between ultrasound and contrast media. As a result, "contrast-specific" hardware and software systems have been introduced by different ultrasound manufacturers with impressive speed. This has finally led to the birth of a very new imaging modality – "contrast-enhanced sonography" (CEUS).

Since 1999, the introduction of second-generation contrast agents has represented a decisive step towards the extensive clinical use of CEUS and has simultaneously made obsolete most, if not all, scientific publications available so far. This book is, to our knowledge, the first to deal entirely with second-generation contrast agents and the most updated contrast-specific software for noncardiologic uses.

The reasons why the liver has been chosen as the only "target" of the book are easily understandable by radiologists and hepatologists alike. The study of vascularity is the only purpose of CEUS, and the liver has a unique vascular system, with two different inflow systems resulting in a single outflow. Furthermore, the pathologically different focal liver lesions (FLLs) are mostly characterized by different "models" of vascularity: CEUS can mimic contrast-enhanced computed tomography and magnetic resonance imaging, basing differential diagnosis on the morphological and temporal characteristics of enhancement, but with the additional unique advantage of the study being done in real-time.

Technological aspects of contrast agents and related sonographic hardware and software are described in the first chapters of the book. In the clinical sections, the outstanding concepts of liver physiology (mostly vascular) are reviewed and the vascular patterns of various types of FLLs are described, in correlation with histopathology and clinical data. The implications derived from the addition of CEUS to other imaging modalities currently employed are discussed chapter by chapter and completed with considerations on the diagnostic work-up of each type of FLL. In the "hands-on" section, with extremely practical suggestions, an explanation is given on how this new imaging modality can be used to fulfill the needs of radiologists, hepatologists, and oncologists. Being a new modality, it is also important to be aware of the major pitfalls of CEUS and to "adapt" its technique to different clinical situations, with knowledge of various tips and tricks: all this is summarized in the final chapters.

This text is the result of the collaboration of a group of "pioneers" of CEUS who, continuously exchanging new ideas and experiences, have also progressively increased their friendly relationships. Unfortunately, the very first pioneer of the group, our great friend Albrecht, is no longer with us: we will always miss his valuable professional contributions and, more importantly, his friendship.

Contents

Contributors

LUCA AIANI
Servizio di Radiologia
Ospedale Valduce
Via Dante 11
22100 Como, Italy

ALBRECHT BAUER[†]
Bracco Diagnostics Inc.
Princeton, NJ, USA

DIRK BECKER
Chairman, Dept. of Medicine
Gastroenterology, Intensive Care
Medicine
Eckernförde Community Hospital
Schleswiger Str. 114 - 116
D-24340 Eckernförde, Germany

ANDREA BELLOBUONO
Dept. of Radiology
General Hospital
Piazzale Solaro 3
21052 Busto Arsizio (VA), Italy

CLAUDIA BORGHI
Servizio di Radiologia
Ospedale Valduce
Via Dante 11
22100 Como, Italy

PETER N. BURNS
Depts. of Medical Biophysics and
Radiology
University of Toronto
Sunnybrook and Women's Health
Sciences Centre
Toronto, Canada

JEAN MICHEL CORREAS
Service de Radiologie Adulte
Hôpital Necker Enfants Malades
149 rue de Sèvres
75743 Paris Cédex 15, France

LUCA COVA
Dept. of Radiology
General Hospital
Piazzale Solaro 3
21052 Busto Arsizio (VA), Italy

O. HÉLÉNON
Service de Radiologie Adulte
Hôpital Necker Enfants Malades
149 rue de Sèvres
75743 Paris Cédex 15, France

VALENTINA KIRN
Dept. of Radiology
General Hospital
Piazzale Solaro 3
21052 Busto Arsizio (VA), Italy

EDWARD LEEN
Consultant Radiologist/Senior Lecturer
University of Glasgow
Dept. of Radiology
Royal Infirmary
Alexandra Parade
Glasgow G31 2ER, UK

ALBERTO MARTEGANI
Servizio di Radiologia
Ospedale Valduce
Via Dante 11
22100 Como, Italy

VALERIA OSTI
Dept. of Radiology
General Hospital
Piazzale Solaro 3
21052 Busto Arsizio (VA), Italy

LUIGI SOLBIATI
Chairman, Dept. of Radiology
General Hospital
Piazzale Solaro 3
21052 Busto Arsizio (VA), Italy

MASSIMO TONOLINI
Dept. of Radiology
General Hospital
Piazzale Solaro 3
21052 Busto Arsizio (VA), Italy

1 Contrast Ultrasound Technology

P.N. Burns

1.1
Introduction: The Need for Bubble-Specific Imaging

One of the major diagnostic objectives in using an ultrasound contrast agent in the liver is to detect flow in the circulation at a level that is lower than would otherwise be possible. The echoes from blood associated with such flow – in the sinusoids for example – exist in the midst of echoes from the surrounding solid structures of the liver parenchyma, echoes which are almost always stronger than even the contrast-enhanced blood echo. When they can be seen, blood vessels in a nonenhanced image have a low echo level, so that an echo-enhancing agent actually *lowers* the contrast between blood and the surrounding tissue, making the lumen of the blood vessel less visible. Thus, in order to be able to image flow in small vessels of the liver, a contrast agent is required that either enhances the blood echo to a level that is substantially higher than that of the surrounding tissue, or can be used with a method for suppressing the echo from non-contrast-bearing structures. X-ray angiography, which is faced with a similar problem, deals with these 'clutter' components of the image by simple subtraction of a preinjection image. What is left behind might reveal flow in individual vessels or the 'blush' of perfusion at the tissue level. If, however, we subtract two consecutive ultrasound images of an abdominal organ, we are likely to get a third ultrasound image, produced by the shift or *decorrelation* of the speckle pattern between acquisitions. In order to show parenchymal enhancement, speckle variance must first be re-duced by filtering, with an unacceptable loss of spatial or temporal resolution. Even if the speckle problem could be overcome, subtraction would still be poorly suited to the dynamic and interactive nature of ultrasound imaging.

Doppler is an alternative method that successfully separates echoes from blood and tissue. It relies on the relatively high velocity of blood compared to that of the surrounding tissue. Although this distinction – which allows us to use a highpass (or 'wall') filter to separate the Doppler signals due to blood flow from those due to clutter – is valid for flow in large vessels, it does not work for flow at the parenchymal level, where the tissue is moving at the same speed or faster than the blood which perfuses it. In this case the Doppler shift frequency from the moving solid tissue is comparable to or higher than that of the moving blood itself. Furthermore, the amplitude of the solid tissue echo is typically more than 10,000 times higher than that of the blood echo. Because the wall filter cannot be used without eliminating both the flow and the clutter echoes, the use of Doppler in such circumstances is defeated by the overwhelming signal from tissue movement: the 'flash' artifact in colour or the 'thump' artifact in spectral Doppler. Thus, true parenchymal flow cannot be imaged using conventional Doppler, with or without intravenous contrast agents (Fig. 1.1).

How then might contrast agents be used to improve the visibility of small vascular structures within tissue? Clearly, a method that could identify the echo from the contrast agent and thereby suppress that from solid tissue would provide both a real-time 'subtraction'

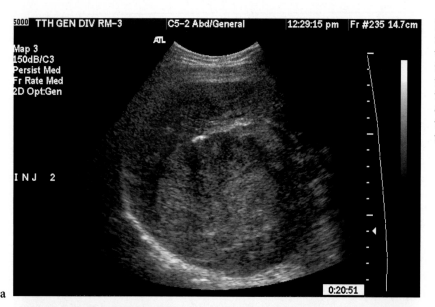

a

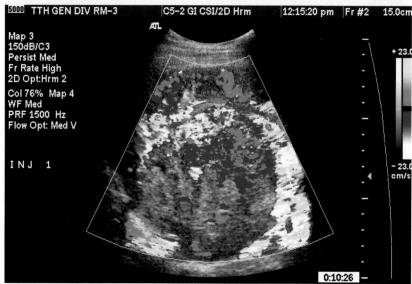

b

Fig. 1.1 a, b. The need for contrast-specific imaging. **a** Conventional image of liver containing large mass. **b** Administration of contrast increases the echogenicity of blood but creates Doppler artifacts due to blooming and tissue motion. (From *Burns et al. 2000*)

mode for contrast-enhanced B-mode imaging, and a means of suppressing Doppler clutter without the use of a velocity-dependent filter in spectral and colour modes. Contrast-specific imaging (often referred to as *nonlinear* imaging) aims to provide such a method, and hence the means for the detection of flow in smaller vessels than is currently possible.

1.1.1
Bubble Behaviour and Incident Pressure

The key to understanding contrast imaging instruments – and the key to their successful clinical use – lies in the unique interaction between a microbubble contrast agent and the process that images them. Controlling and exploiting this interaction is central to all contrast-specific methods. Unlike tissue, contrast microbubbles scatter ultrasound in a manner dependent on the amplitude of the sound to which they are exposed by the imaging process. There are three broad regimes of scattering behaviour that depend on the peak pressure of the incident sound field produced by the scanner. These form the basis of contrast imaging methods for the liver. At low incident pressures (corresponding to low transmit power of the scanner), the agents produce linear backscatter enhancement, resulting in an augmentation of the echo from blood. This is the behaviour originally envisaged by contrast agent manufacturers for their first intended clinical indication: Doppler signal enhancement. As the transmit intensity control of the scanner is increased and the pressure incident on a bubble goes beyond about 50-100 kPa, which is still below the level used in most diagnostic scans, the contrast agent backscatter begins to show nonlinear characteristics, such as the emission of harmonics. It is the detection of these harmonics that forms the basis of contrast-specific imaging modes such as harmonic and pulse inversion imaging and Doppler. Finally, as the peak pressure reaches 1 MPa, near the maximum emitted by a typical ultrasound imaging system, many agents exhibit transient nonlinear scattering, resulting in their destruction. This forms the basis of triggered imaging and the most sensitive methods for detecting perfusion. It should be noted that in practice, because of the different sizes present in a realistic population of bubbles (*Chin and Burns 1997*), the borders between these behaviours are not sharp. Nor will they be the same for different agent types, whose acoustic behaviour is strongly dependent on the gas and shell properties (*de Jong 1997*).

1.1.2
The Mechanical Index

For reasons unrelated to contrast imaging, ultrasound scanners marketed in the USA are required by the Food and Drugs Administration (FDA) to carry an on-screen label of the estimated peak negative pressure to which tissue is exposed. Of course, this pressure changes according to the tissue through which the sound travels as well as the amplitude and geometry of the ultrasound beam: the higher the attenuation, the less the peak pressure in tissue will be. A scanner cannot 'know' what tissue it is being used on, so the definition of an index has been arrived at which reflects the approximate exposure to ultrasound pressure at the focus of the beam in an average tissue. The mechanical index (or MI) is defined as the peak rarefactional (that is, negative) pressure, divided by the square root of the ultrasound frequency.

This quantity is related to the amount of mechanical work that can be performed on a bubble during a single negative half cycle of sound (*Apfel and Holland 1991*). In clinical ultrasound systems, this index usually lies somewhere between 0.1 and 2.0. Although a single value is displayed for each image, in practice the actual MI varies throughout the image. In the absence of attenuation, the MI is maximal at the focus of the beam. Attenuation shifts this maximum towards the transducer. Furthermore, because it is a somewhat complex procedure to calculate the index, which is itself only an estimate of the actual quantity within the body, the indices displayed by different machines are not precisely comparable. Thus, for example, more bubble disruption might be observed at a displayed MI of 1.0 using one machine than on the same patient using another. For this reason, recommendations of machine settings for a specific examination are not transferable between manufacturers' instruments. Nonetheless, the MI is one of the most important machine parameters in a contrast study. It is usually controlled by means of the "output power" control of the scanner.

1.2
Nonlinear Backscatter: Harmonic Imaging

Examining the behaviour of contrast-enhanced ultrasound studies reveals two important pieces of evidence. First, the size of the echo enhancement at very high dilution following a small peripheral injection [7 dB from as little as 0.01 ml/kg of Levovist®, for example (*Burns et al. 1994*)] is much larger than would be expected from such sparse scatterers of this size in blood. Second, investigations of the acoustic characteristics of several agents (*Bleeker et al. 1990*) have demonstrated peaks in the spectra of attenuation and scattering which are dependent on both ultrasound frequency and the size of the microbubbles. This important observation suggests that the bubbles *resonate* in an ultrasound field. As the ultrasound wave – which comprises alternate compressions and rarefactions – propagates

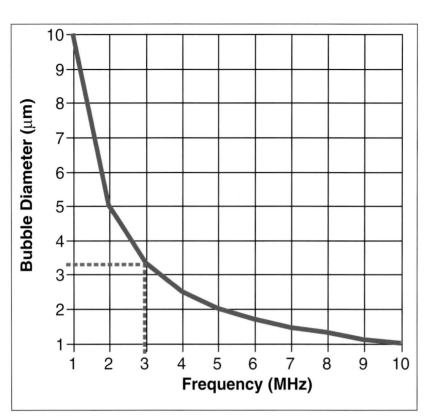

Fig. 1.2. Microbubbles resonate in a diagnostic ultrasound field. This graph shows that the resonant – or natural – frequency of oscillation of a bubble of air in an ultrasound field depends on its size. For a 3.5-µm diameter, the size needed for an intravenously injectible contrast agent, the resonant frequency is about 3 MHz

over the bubbles, they experience a periodic change in their radius in sympathy with the oscillations of the incident sound. Like vibrations in other structures, these radial oscillations have a natural – or *resonant* – frequency of oscillation at which they will both absorb and scatter ultrasound with a peculiarly high efficiency. Considering the linear oscillation of a free bubble of air in water, we can use a simple theory (*Ophir and Parker 1989*) to predict the resonant frequency of radial oscillation of a bubble of 3 µm diameter, the median diameter of a typical transpulmonary microbubble agent. As Fig. 1.2 shows, it is about 3 MHz, approximately the centre frequency of ultrasound used in a typical abdominal scan. This extraordinary – and fortunate – coincidence explains why ultrasound contrast agents are so efficient and can be administered in such small quantities. It also predicts that bubbles undergoing resonant oscillation in an ultrasound field can be induced to nonlinear motion, the basis of harmonic imaging.

It has long been recognised (*Neppiras et al. 1983*) that if bubbles are 'driven' by an ultrasound field at sufficiently high acoustic pressures, the oscillatory excursions of the bubble reach a point where the alternate expansions and contractions of the bubble's size are not equal. Lord Rayleigh, the originator of the theoretical understanding of sound upon which ultrasound imaging is based, was first led in 1917 to investigate this by his curiosity over the creaking noises that his tea-kettle made as the water came to the boil. The consequence of such nonlinear motion is that the sound emitted by the bubble, and detected by the transducer, contains harmonics, just as the resonant strings of a musical instrument, if plucked too vigorously, will produce a 'harsh' timbre containing overtones (the musical term for harmonics) exact octaves above the fundamental note. The origin of this phenomenon is the asymmetry which begins to affect bubble oscillation as the amplitude becomes large. As a bubble is compressed by the ultrasound pressure wave, it becomes stiffer and hence resists further reduction in its radius. Conversely, in the rarefaction phase of the ultrasound pulse, the bubble becomes less stiff, and, therefore, enlarges much more (Fig. 1.3). Figure 1.4 shows the frequency spectrum of an echo produced

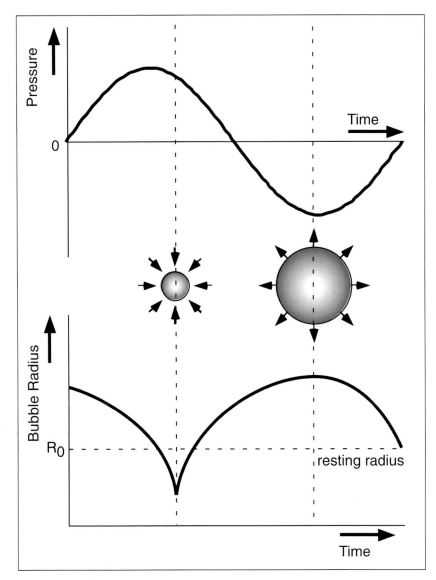

Fig. 1.3. A microbubble in an acoustic field. Bubbles respond asymmetrically to high-intensity sound waves, stiffening when compressed by sound, yielding only small changes in radius. During the low-pressure portion of the sound wave, the bubble stiffness decreases and radius changes can be large. This asymmetric response leads to the production of harmonics in the scattered wave

by a microbubble contrast agent following a 3.75-MHz burst. The particular agent is Levovist, although many microbubble agents behave in a similar way. Ultrasound frequency is on the horizontal axis, with the relative amplitude on the vertical axis. A strong echo, at -13 dB with respect to the fundamental, is seen at twice the transmitted frequency, that known as the second harmonic. Peaks in the echo spectrum at sub- and ultraharmonics are also seen. Here, then, is one simple method to distinguish bubbles from tissue: excite them so as to produce harmonics and detect these in preference to the fundamental echo from tissue. Key factors in the harmonic response of an agent, which varies from material to material,

are the incident pressure of the ultrasound field, the frequency, as well as the size distribution of the bubbles and the mechanical properties of the bubble capsule (a stiff capsule, for example, will dampen the oscillations and attenuate the nonlinear response).

1.2.1
Harmonic B-Mode Imaging

An imaging and Doppler method based on this principle, called harmonic imaging (*Burns et al. 1992*), is now widely available on most modern ultrasound scanners. In harmonic mode, the system transmits normally at one frequency, but is tuned to receive echoes preferentially

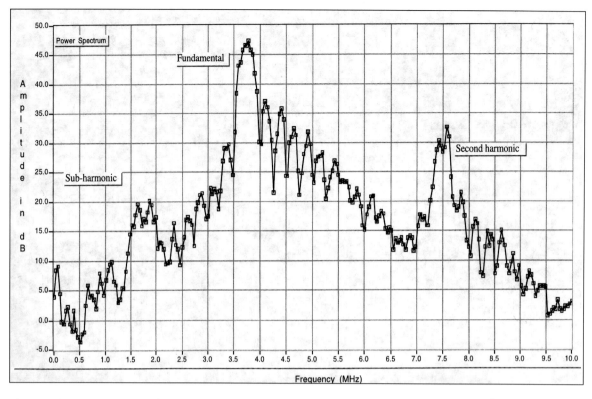

Fig. 1.4. Harmonic emission from Levovist®. A sample of a contrast agent is insonated at 3.75 MHz and the echo analyzed for its frequency content. It is seen that most of the energy in the echo is at 3.75 MHz, but that there is a clear second peak in the spectrum at 7.5 MHz, as well as a third at 1.875 MHz. The second harmonic echo is only 13 dB less than that of the main, or fundamental echo. Harmonic imaging and Doppler aim to separate and process this signal alone. The smaller peak is the first subharmonic. (From *Becher and Burns 2000*)

at double that frequency, where the echoes from the bubbles lie. Typically, the transmit frequency lies between 1.5 and 3 MHz and the receive frequency is selected by means of a bandpass filter whose centre frequency is at the second harmonic between 3 and 6 MHz. Harmonic imaging uses the same array transducers as conventional imaging and for most of today's ultrasound systems involves only software changes. Echoes from solid tissue, as well as red blood cells themselves, are suppressed. Real-time harmonic spectral Doppler and colour Doppler modes have also been implemented (sometimes experimentally) on a number of commercially available systems. Clearly, an exceptional transducer bandwidth is needed to operate over such a large range of frequencies. Fortunately much effort has been directed in recent years towards increasing the bandwidth of transducer arrays because of its significant bearing on conventional imaging

performance, so harmonic imaging modes do not require the additional expense of dedicated transducers.

1.2.2
Harmonic Doppler

In harmonic images, the echo from tissue-mimicking material is reduced – but not eliminated –, reversing the contrast between the agent and its surrounding (Fig. 1.5b). The value of this effect is to increase the conspicuity of the agent when it is in blood vessels normally hidden by the strong echoes from tissue. In spectral Doppler, one would expect the suppression of the tissue echo to reduce the tissue motion 'thump' that is familiar to all Doppler sonographers. Figure 1.6 shows spectral Doppler applied to a region of the aorta in which there is wall motion as well as blood flow within the sample volume. The conven-

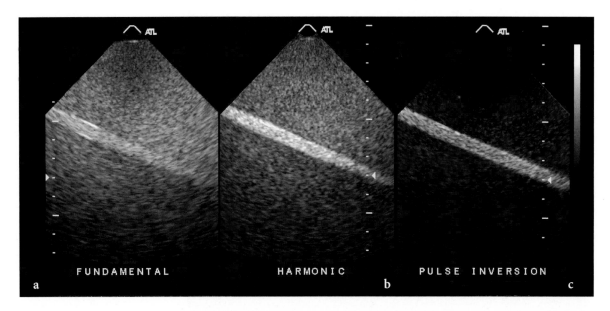

Fig. 1.5 a-c. Demostration of pulse inversion imaging. In vitro images of a vessel phantom containing stationary contrast agent (Optison®) surrounded by tissue-equivalent material (biogel and graphite). **a** Conventional image, MI = 0.2. **b** Harmonic imaging, MI = 0.2, provides improved contrast between agent and tissue. **c** Pulse inversion imaging, MI = 0.2. By suppressing linear echoes from stationary tissue, pulse inversion imaging provides better contrast between agent and tissue than both conventional and harmonic imaging. (From *Becher and Burns 2000*)

tional Doppler image of Figure 1.7a shows the thump artifact due to clutter, which is almost completely absent in the harmonic Doppler image of Figure 1.7b (all instrument settings, including the filters, are identical). In vivo measurements from spectral Doppler show that the signal-to-clutter ratio is improved by a combination of harmonic imaging and the contrast agent by as much as 35 dB (*Burns et al. 1993*). Applications of this method include detection of blood flow in small vessels surrounded by tissue which is moving: the branches of the coronary arteries (*Mulvagh et al. 1996*), the myocardium itself (*Porter et al. 1996*), as well as in the parenchyma of abdominal organs (*Kono et al. 1996*).

1.2.3
Harmonic Power Doppler Imaging

In colour Doppler studies using a contrast agent, the effect of the arrival of the agent in a colour region of interest is often to produce blooming of the colour image, whereby signals from major vascular targets spread out to occupy the entire region. Although flow from

smaller vessels might be detectable, the colour images can be swamped by artifactual signals. (Fig. 1.1b). The origin of this artifact is the amplitude thresholding that governs most colour displays in conventional (or 'velocity') mode imaging. Increasing the backscattered signal power simply has the effect of displaying the velocity estimate, at full intensity, over a wider range of pixels around the detected location. A display in which the parameter mapped to colour is related directly to the backscattered signal power, on the other hand, has the advantage that such thresholding is unnecessary and that lower amplitude Doppler shifts, such as those which result from sidelobe interference, are displayed at a lower visual amplitude, rendering them less conspicuous. Echo-enhanced flow signals, in contrast, will be displayed at a higher level. This is the basis of the *Doppler power imaging* (also known as *colour power angiography*, or *colour Doppler energy* mapping). Power Doppler can help eliminate some other limitations of small vessel flow detection with colour Doppler. Low-velocity detection requires lowering the Doppler pulse repetition frequency (PRF), which results in multiple

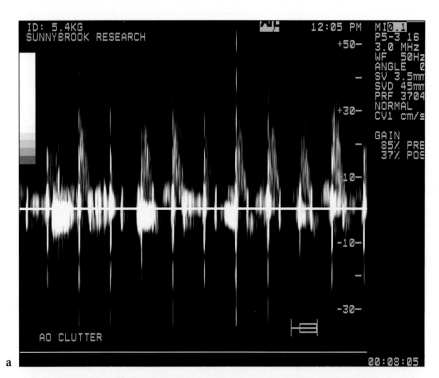

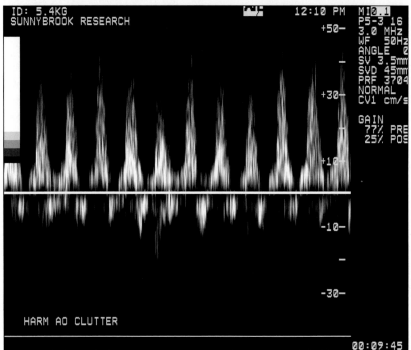

Fig. 1.6 a,b. Clutter rejection with harmonic spectral Doppler. **a** The abdominal aorta is examined with harmonic spectral Doppler. In conventional mode, clutter from the moving wall causes the familiar artifact which also obscures diastolic flow. **b** In harmonic mode, the clutter is almost completely suppressed, so that flow can be resolved. The settings of the filter and other relevant instrument parameters are identical. (From *Becher and Burns 2000*)

aliasing and loss of directional resolution. A display method that does not use the velocity estimate is not prone to the aliasing artifact, and therefore allows the PRF to be lowered and hence increases the likelihood of detection of the lower velocity flow from smaller vessels.

Because it maps a parameter directly related to the acoustic quantity that is enhanced by the contrast agent, the power map is a natural choice for contrast-enhanced colour Doppler studies. However, the advantages of the power map for contrast-enhanced detection of small

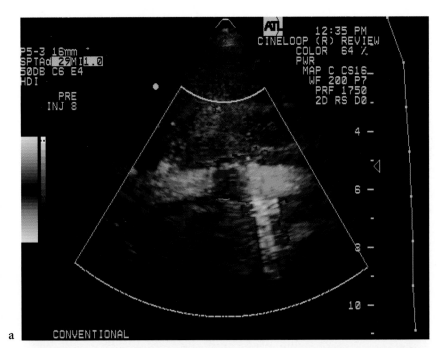

Fig. 1.7 a,b. Reduction of the flash artifact in harmonic power Doppler. The harmonic contrast method helps overcome one of the principal shortcomings of power Doppler, its increased susceptibility to tissue motion. **a** Aortic flow in power mode with flash artifact from cardiac motion of the wall. **b** In harmonic mode at the same point in the cardiac cycle, the flash is largely suppressed. All instrument settings are the same. (From *Becher and Burns 2000*)

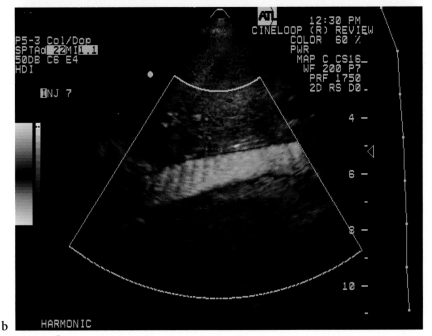

vessel flow are balanced by a potentially devastating shortcoming: its increased susceptibility to interference from clutter. Clutter is both detected more readily, because of the power mode's increased sensitivity, and displayed more prominently, because of the high-intensity display of high-amplitude signals. Furthermore, frame averaging has the additional effect of sustaining and blurring the flash over the cardiac cycle, thus exacerbating its effect on the image. This is the reason that conventional power mode, while quite popular in some organ imaging, has no application where there is tissue motion.

At the small expense of some sensitivity, amply compensated by the enhancement caused by the agent, harmonic mode effectively overcomes this clutter problem (Fig. 1.7). Combining the harmonic method with power Doppler produces an especially effective tool for the detection of flow in the small vessels of the organs of the abdomen which may be moving with cardiac pulsation or respiration. In a study in which flow imaged on contrast-enhanced power harmonic images was compared with histologically sized arterioles in the corresponding regions of the renal cortex (*Burns et al. 1994*), it was concluded that the method is capable of demonstrating flow in vessels of less than 40 μm diameter; about ten times smaller than the corresponding imaging resolution limit, even as the organ was moving with normal respiration. Using this power mode method in the heart, flow can be imaged in the myocardium (*Burns et al. 1996a; Becher 1997*).

1.2.4
Tissue Harmonic Imaging

In second harmonic imaging, an ultrasound scanner transmits at one frequency and receives at double this frequency. The resulting improved detection of the microbubble echo is due to the peculiar behaviour of a gas bubble in an ultrasound field. However, any source of a received signal at the harmonic frequency which does not come from the bubble will clearly reduce the efficacy of this method. Such unwanted signals can come from nonlinearities in the transducer or its associated electronics, and these must be tackled effectively in a good harmonic imaging system. However, tissue itself can produce harmonics which will be received by the transducer. They are developed as a wave *propagates* through tissue. Again, this is due to an asymmetry: this time, the fact that sound travels slightly faster through tissue during the compressional part of the cycle (where it is denser and hence more stiff) than during the rarefactional part. Although the effect is very small, it is sufficient to produce substantial harmonic components in the transmitted wave by the time it reaches deep tissue, so that when it is scattered by a linear target such as the myocardium, there is a harmonic component in the echo, which is detected by the scanner along with the harmonic echo from the bubble (*Hamilton and Blackstock 1998*). This is why solid tissue is not com-

pletely dark in a typical harmonic image. The effect is to reduce the contrast between the bubble and tissue, rendering the problem of detecting perfusion in tissue more difficult.

Tissue harmonics, although a foe to contrast imaging, are not necessarily a bad thing. In fact, an image formed from tissue harmonics without the presence of contrast agents has many properties which recommend it over conventional imaging. These come from the fact that tissue harmonics are developed as the beam penetrates tissue, in contrast to the conventional beam, which is generated at the transducer surface (*Becher and Burns 2000*). Artifacts which accrue from the first few centimetres of tissue, such as reverberations, are reduced by using tissue harmonic imaging. Sidelobe and other low-level interference is also suppressed, making tissue harmonic imaging the routine modality of choice for many sonographers.

Nonetheless, for contrast studies, the tissue harmonic limits the visibilty of bubbles within tissue and therefore can be considered an artifact. In considering how to reduce it, it is instructive to bear in mind differences between harmonics produced by tissue propagation and by bubble echoes. First, tissue harmonics require a high peak pressure, so are only evident at high MI. Reducing the MI leaves only the bubble harmonics. Second, harmonics from tissue at high MI are continuous and sustained, whereas those from bubbles at high MI are transient in nature as the bubble disrupts.

1.2.5
Pulse Inversion Imaging

Harmonic imaging imposes some fundamental limitations on the imaging process which restrict its clinical potential in organ imaging. First, in order to ensure that the higher frequencies are due only to harmonics emitted by the bubbles, the transmitter must be restricted to a band of frequencies around the fundamental (Fig. 1.8a). Similarly, the received band of frequencies must be restricted to those lying around the second harmonic. If these two regions overlap (Fig. 1.8b), the result will be that the harmonic filter will receive echoes from ordinary tissue, thus reducing the contrast be-

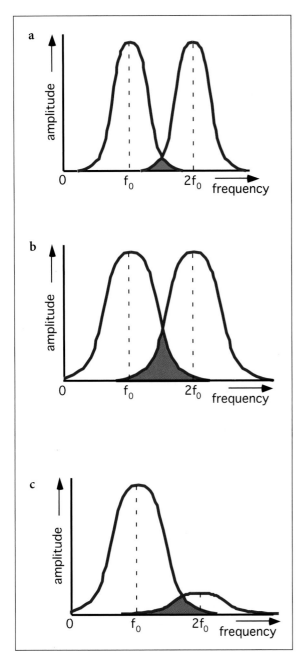

Fig. 1.8 a-c. The compromises forced by harmonic imaging. **a** In harmonic imaging, the transmitted frequencies must be restricted to a band around the fundamental , and the receive frequencies must be limited to a band around the second harmonic. This limits resolution. **b** If the transmit and receive bandwidths are increased to improve resolution, some fundamental echoes from tissue will overlap the receive bandwidth and will be detected, reducing contrast between agent and tissue. **c** When the harmonic echoes are weak, due to low agent concentration and/or low incident pulse intensity, this overlap will be especially large, and the harmonic signal may be largely composed of tissue echoes

tween the agent and tissue. However, restricting the receive bandwidth degrades the resolution of the resulting image, thus framing a fundamental compromise in harmonic imaging between contrast and resolution. For optimal detection of bubbles in the microvasculature, this compromise must favour contrast, so that the most sensitive harmonic images are generally of low quality. A further drawback of the filtering approach is that if the received echo is weak, the overlapping region between the transmit and receive frequencies becomes a larger portion of the entire received signal (Fig. 1.8c). Thus contrast in the harmonic image is dependent on how strong the echo is from the bubbles, which is determined by the concentration of bubbles and the intensity of the incident ultrasound pulse. In practice, this forces use of a high MI in harmonic mode, resulting in the transient and irreversible disruption of the bubbles (*Burns et al. 1996b*). As the bubbles enter the scan plane of a real-time ultrasound image, they provide an echo but then disappear. Thus vessels that lie within the scan plane are not visualized as continuous ducts in a typical harmonic image; but instead have a punctate appearance (Fig. 1.9a).

1.2.5.1
Principle of Pulse Inversion

Pulse inversion imaging overcomes the conflict between the requirements of contrast and resolution in harmonic imaging and provides greater sensitivity, thus allowing low incident power, nondestructive, continuous imaging of microbubbles in an organ such as the liver. The method also relies on the asymmetric oscillation of an ultrasound bubble in an acoustic field, but detects 'even' nonlinear components of the echo over the entire bandwidth of the transducer. In pulse inversion (also known as phase inversion) imaging, two pulses are sent in rapid succession into the tissue. The second pulse is a mirror image of the first (Fig. 1.10): that is, it has undergone a 180° phase change. The scanner detects the echo from these two successive pulses and forms their sum. For ordinary tissue, which behaves in a linear manner, the sum of two inverted pulses is simply zero. For an echo with nonlinear components,

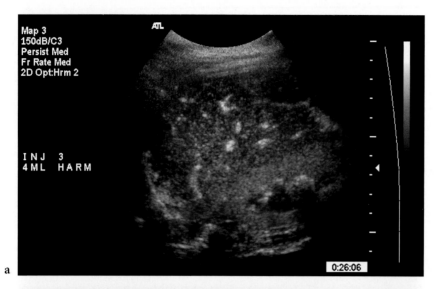

a

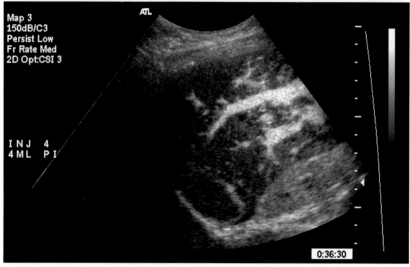

b

Fig. 1.9 a,b. The appearance of blood vessels in harmonic and pulse inversion imaging in a study patient with an incidental haemangioma (From *Becher and Burns 2000*). **a** In a harmonic contrast image of a liver, large vessels have a punctate appearance as the high MI ultrasound disrupts the bubbles as they enter the scan plane. **b** In the pulse inversion image of the same liver, a lower MI can be used so that continuous vessels are now seen. Improved resolution of pulse inversion imaging demonstrates fourth order branches of the portal vein

such as that from a bubble, the echoes produced from these two pulses will not be simple mirror images of each other, because of the asymmetric behaviour of the bubble radius with time. The result is that the sum of these two echoes is not zero. Thus, a signal is detected from a bubble but not from tissue. It can be shown mathematically that this summed echo contains the nonlinear even harmonic components of the signal, including the second harmonic (*Hope Simpson et al. 1999*). One advantage of pulse inversion over the filter approach to detect harmonics from bubbles is that it no longer suffers from the restriction of bandwidth. The full frequency range of sound emitted from the transducer can be detected in this way, providing a full bandwidth, that is high

resolution, image of the echoes from bubbles (*Burns et al. 2000*). Figure 1.5c illustrates how pulse inversion imaging provides better suppression of linear echoes than harmonic imaging and is effective over the full bandwidth of the transducer, showing improvement of image resolution over harmonic mode. Because this detection method is a more efficient means of isolating the bubble echo, weaker echoes from bubbles insonated at low, nondestructive intensities can be detected. Figure 1.9b shows a pulse inversion imaging of the same liver as Figure 1.9a, at low MI. Fourth order branches of the portal vein are visible. It should be noted, however, that as the MI increases, tissue harmonic renders the tissue brighter. Indeed pulse inversion is now the preferred method

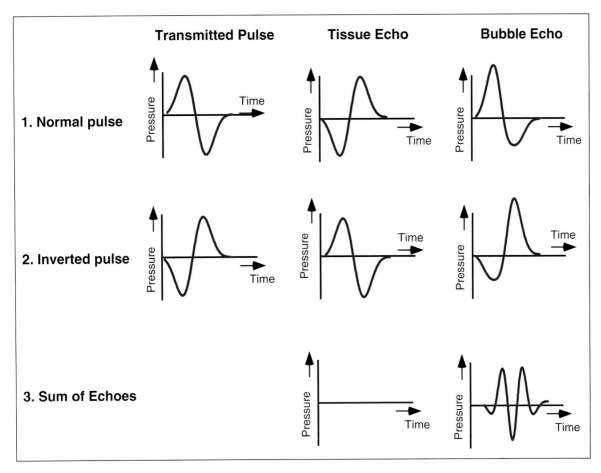

Fig. 1.10. Basic principle of pulse inversion imaging. A pulse of sound is transmitted into the body and echoes are received from agent and tissue. A second pulse, which is an inverted copy of the first pulse, is then transmitted in the same direction and the two echoes are summed. Linear echoes from tissue will be inverted copies of each other and will cancel to zero. The microbubble echoes are distorted copies of each other, and the nonlinear components of these echoes will reinforce each other when summed, producing a strong harmonic signal. (From *Becher and Burns 2000*)

used by many systems for tissue harmonic imaging. Optimal pulse inversion contrast imaging is often, then, performed at low MI.

1.2.6
Power Pulse Inversion Imaging

In spite of the improvements offered by pulse inversion over harmonic imaging for suppressing stationary tissue, the method is somewhat sensitive to echoes from moving tissue. This is because tissue motion causes linear echoes to change slightly between pulses, so that they do not cancel perfectly. Furthermore, at high MI, nonlinear propagation also causes harmonic echoes to appear in pulse inversion images, even from linear scattering structures such as

the liver parenchyma. While tissue motion artifacts can be minimized by using a short pulse repetition interval, nonlinear tissue echoes can mask the echoes from bubbles, reducing the efficacy of microbubble contrast, especially when a high MI is used. A recent development seeks to address these problems by means of a generalization of the pulse inversion method, called pulse inversion Doppler (*Hope Simpson et al. 1999*). This technique – which is also known as *power pulse inversion imaging* – combines the nonlinear detection performance of pulse inversion imaging with the motion discrimination capabilities of power Doppler. Multiple transmit pulses of alternating polarity are used and Doppler signal processing techniques are

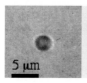   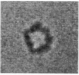

5 µm

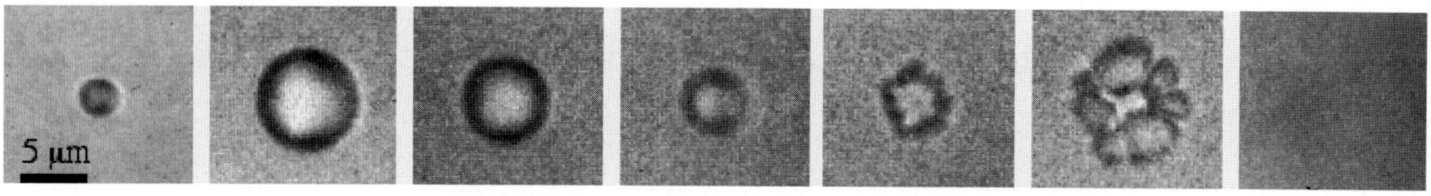

Fig. 1.11. Fragmentation of contrast agent observed with a high-speed camera by researchers at the University of California, Davis. The frame images are captured over 50 ns. The bubble is insonated with 2.4 MHz ultrasound with a peak negative pressure of 1.1 MPa (MI~0.7). The bubble is initially 3 µm in diameter and fragments during compression after the first expansion. Resulting bubble fragments are not seen after insonation, because they are either fully dissolved or below the optical resolution. (From *Becher and Burns 2000*)

applied to distinguish between bubble echoes and echoes from moving tissue and/or tissue harmonics, as desired by the operator. This method offers potential improvements in the agent-to-tissue contrast and signal-to-noise performance, although at the cost of a somewhat reduced framerate. The most dramatic manifestation of this method's ability to detect very weak harmonic echoes has been its first demonstration of real-time perfusion imaging of the myocardium (*Tiemann et al. 1999*). By lowering the MI to 0.1 or less, bubbles undergo stable, nonlinear oscillation, emitting continuous harmonic signals. Because of the low MI, very few bubbles are disrupted, so that imaging can take place at real-time rates. Because sustained, stable nonlinear oscillation is required for this method, perfluorocarbon gas bubbles work best.

1.3
Transient Disruption: Intermittent Imaging

As the incident pressure to which a resonating bubble is exposed increases, so its oscillation becomes more wild, with the radius increasing in some bubbles by a factor of five or more during the rarefaction phase of the incident sound. Just as a resonating violin string, if bowed over-zealously, will break, so a microbubble, if driven by intense ultrasound, will suffer irreversible disruption of its shell. A physical picture of precisely what happens to a disrupted bubble is only now emerging from high-speed video studies (*Dayton et al. 1999*). It is certain, however, that the bubble disappears as an acoustic scatterer (not instantly,

but over a period of time determined by the bubble composition), and that as it does so it emits a strong, brief nonlinear echo. It is this echo whose detection is the basis of the most sensitive method for detecting microbubble contrast at the perfusion level.

1.3.1
Triggered Imaging

It was discovered during the early days of harmonic imaging that by pressing the 'freeze' button on a scanner for a few moments, and hence interrupting the acquisition of ultrasound images during a contrast study, it is possible to increase the effectiveness of a contrast agent. So dramatic is this effect that it was responsible for the first ultrasound images of myocardial perfusion using harmonic imaging (*Porter and Xie 1995*). This is a consequence of the ability of the ultrasound field, if its peak pressure is sufficiently high, to disrupt a bubble's shell and hence destroy it (*Burns et al. 1996b; Uhlendorf and Scholle 1996*) (Fig. 1.11). As the bubble is disrupted, it releases energy, so creating a strong, transient echo, which is rich in harmonics. This process is sometimes incorrectly referred to as "stimulated acoustic emission". The fact that this echo is transient in nature can be exploited for its detection. One simple method is to subtract from a disruption image a baseline image obtained either before or (more usefully) immediately after insonation. Such a method requires offline processing of stored ultrasound images, together with software which can align the ultrasound images before subtraction, and is only useful in rare circumstances (*Becher and Burns 2000*).

1.3.2
Intermittent Harmonic Power Doppler for Perfusion Imaging

Power Doppler imaging was described earlier as a technique designed to detect the motion of blood or of tissue. It works by a simple, pulse-to-pulse subtraction method (*Taylor et al. 1996*), in which two or more pulses are sent successively along each scan line of the image. Pairs of received echo trains are compared for each line: if they are identical, nothing is displayed, but if there is a change (due to motion of the tissue between pulses), a colour is displayed whose saturation is related to the amplitude of the echo that has changed. This method, although not designed for the detection of bubble disruption, is ideally suited for high MI destruction imaging. The first pulse receives an echo from the bubble, the second receives none, so the comparison yields a strong signal. In a sense, power Doppler may be thought of as a line-by-line subtraction procedure on the radiofrequency echo detected by the transducer. Interestingly for liver scanning, pulse inversion imaging – the most commonly used method at low MI – becomes equivalent to power Doppler if the MI is high and the bubble disrupted. Looking at Figure 1.9, one can easily see that if the echo from the second pulse is absent (because the bubble is gone), the sum of the two bubble echoes is the same as their difference, which is what is measured by power Doppler. The fact that the second transmitted pulse is inverted is immaterial for the bubble that has disappeared!

One critical question is how long one needs to wait between pulses. If the two pulses are too close together in time, the bubble's gaseous contents, which are dispersed after disruption of the shell by a process of diffusion and fragmentation, will still be able to provide an echo, so reducing the effectiveness of the detection. If the two pulses are too far apart in time, the solid tissue of the myocardium will have moved, so that the detection process will show them as well. There are two solutions. First, by using harmonic detection, some – but not all – of the moving tissue 'clutter' can be rejected. Second, a bubble can be designed to disrupt quickly so that rapid (that is, high PRF) imaging may be used. Such a bubble will have a gas content that is highly diffusible and soluble in blood. In this respect, air is perfect. Diffusion of air after acoustic disruption is about 40 times faster than such diffusion of a perfluorocarbon gas from a similar bubble (*Burns et al. 1996b*), so that air-based agents such as Levovist are the most effective to image in this mode. Nonetheless, very effective imaging of perfluorocarbon bubbles throughout the liver can be made by using a sweep, a method commonly employed to map the distribution of bubbles in the 'postvascular' phase of such agents as SonoVue and Levovist.

This, then, offers two distinct approaches to contrast imaging of the liver, which many investigators now use in combination (*Wilson and Burns 2001*) (Fig. 1.12). A *low MI*, real-time, nondestructive bubble imaging mode can be used to survey vessels in the liver. Such images show tumour vascular morphology and reveal arterialised lesions following a bolus injection of contrast (Fig. 1.12a). The imaging modality of choice here will be pulse inversion [available on various systems as *phase inversion* or *coherent contrast imaging (CCI)*]. Following this examination, a further injection is made and after the agent is seen to enter the hepatic arterial circulation, the scanner is set to *high MI* and frozen for an interval between 5 and 90 s, allowing the agent to enter the hepatic sinusoids. The scanner is unfrozen and a 'flash' or 'veil' is seen as the agent is disrupted (*Wilson et al. 2000*) revealing the entire distribution of bubbles in the liver, including those in the parenchyma. This is a liver 'perfusion' image. Depending on the delay, this can be timed to show the arterial (Fig. 1.12b), portal (Fig. 1.10) or postvascular phases. The preferred modes for this method are pulse inversion – which carries the attraction of high-resolution imaging but the disadvantage of a strong tissue harmonic background – or power Doppler modes such as harmonic power angio or 'agent destruction imaging' (ADI). Many systems now offer a low MI 'monitor' mode that can be used to give a crude (usually fundamental) image of the liver during the interval delay which can be helpful to keep the scanplane aligned in the volume of interest. Pressing a button returns the scanner to the high MI nonlinear mode to produce the 'flash' image of perfusion.

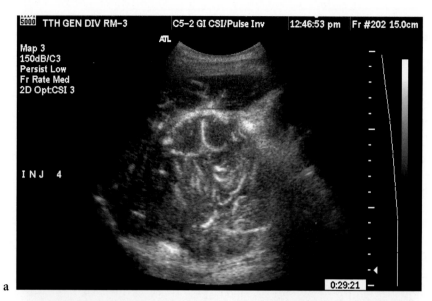

a

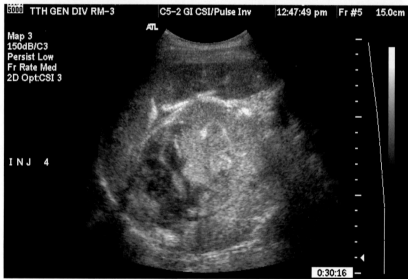

b

Fig. 1.12a, b. Using high and low MI contrast-specific imaging in the same patient as Fig. 1.1. **a** At low MI, real-time pulse inversion imaging reveals the extensive internal vasculature of the lesion, with tortuous vessels defined with a resolution comparable to that of the conventional B-mode image. **b** At high MI, after an 8-s interval delay, arterial perfusion is seen to be present throughout the lesion, with the exception of an area of necrosis, which is well delineated. (From *Burns et al.* 2000)

1.4
Summary

We have defined three behavioural regimes of bubbles in an acoustic field, which depend on the intensity of the transmitted ultrasound beam. In practice, this intensity is best monitored by means of the MI displayed by the scanner. At very low MI, the bubbles act as simple, but powerful echo enhancers. This regime is most useful for spectral Doppler enhancement but is rarely used in the liver. At slightly higher intensities (the bottom of the range of those used diagnostically), the bubbles emit harmonics as they undergo nonlinear oscilla-

tion. These harmonics can be detected by harmonic and pulse inversion imaging, which form the basis of real-time B-mode imaging of vascular structures in the liver. Newer techniques that employ many phase and/or amplitude modulated pulses, such as power pulse inversion (PPI) or contrast pulse sequence (CPS) imaging, are capable of sensitive imaging of perfusion at low MI without disrupting the bubbles. Finally, at the higher intensity setting of the machine used in routine scanning, the bubbles can be disrupted deliberately, emitting a strong, transient echo. Detecting this echo with harmonic power Doppler remains the most sensitive means we have to image bubbles in very low concentration, but it comes at the price of destroying the bubble. Because of the long reperfusion periods of hepatic flow, intermittent imaging using an 'interval delay' in which the high MI imaging is arrested, becomes necessary.

1.5
Safety Considerations

Contrast ultrasound of the liver exposes patients to ultrasound in a way that is identical to that of a normal ultrasound examination. Yet the use of ultrasound pulses to disrupt bubbles which sit in microscopic vessels raises some new questions about the potential for hazard. When a bubble produces the brief echo which is associated with its disruption, it releases energy which it has stored during its exposure to the ultrasound field. Can this energy damage the surrounding tissue? At higher exposure levels, ultrasound is known to produce bioeffects in tissue, the thresholds for which have been studied extensively. Do these thresholds change when bubbles are present in the vasculature? Whereas the safety of ultrasound contrast agents as drugs has been established to the satisfaction of the most stringent requirements of the regulating authorities in a number of countries, it is probably fair to say that there is much to be learned about the interaction between ultrasound and tissue when bubbles are present.

The most extreme of these interactions is known as *cavitation*, which refers to the formation, growth and collapse of a gas cavity in fluid as a result of ultrasound exposure. It has been studied extensively prior to the development of microbubble contrast agents (*Brennan 1995*). In fact, most of the mathematical models used to describe contrast microbubbles were originally developed to model cavitation (*Plesset 1949; Poritsky 1951; Rayleigh 1917*). When sound waves of sufficient intensity travel through a fluid, the rarefactional half-cycle of the sound wave can actually tear the fluid apart, creating spherical cavities within the fluid. The subsequent rapid collapse of these cavities during the compressional half cycle of the sound wave can focus large amounts of energy into a very small volume, raising the temperature at the centre of the collapse to thousands of degrees Kelvin, forming free radicals, and even emitting electromagnetic radiation (*Plesset 1949; Poritsky 1951; Rayleigh 1917*).

The concern over potential cavitation-induced bioeffects in diagnostic ultrasound has led to many experimental studies. With the exception of one which showed cavitation-induced hemorrhage in mouse lung exposed under conditions that differ substantially from those found clinically (*Child et al. 1990*), no evidence of bioeffects from conventional imaging at these levels has been reported. Many more experiments have been made to assess whether the presence of contrast microbubbles can act as cavitation seeds, potentiating bioeffects (*Everbach et al. 1998; Holland et al. 1992; Miller et al. 1997; Miller and Thomas 1995; Miller et al. 1996; Williams et al. 1991*). While more studies have shown that adding contrast agents to blood increased cavitation effects (e.g., peroxide formation, acoustic emissions) and related bioeffects (e.g., hemolysis, platelet lysis), all significant bioeffects occurred with either very high agent concentration, sound pulse duration or MI, or with hematocrit well below the physiological range. In experiments in which clinically relevant values of these parameters have been used (agent concentration <0.2%, pulse duration <2 ms, MI<1.9, hematocrit ~40-45%), no significant bioeffects have been reported to date (*Miller et al. 1997; Uhlendorf and Hoffmann 1994*).

1.6
Conclusion

Unlike contrast agents for other imaging modalities, microbubbles are modified by the process used to image them. Understanding the behaviour of bubbles while exposed to an ultrasound imaging beam is the key to performing an effective contrast ultrasound examination. The appropriate choice of a contrast-specific imaging method is based on the behaviour of the agent and the requirements of the examination. The MI is the major determinant of the response of contrast bubbles to ultrasound. Low MI harmonic and pulse inversion imaging offer real-time B-mode methods for liver vessel imaging. High MI harmonic power Doppler or pulse inversion can be used for intermittent imaging of liver perfusion with contrast agents, while power pulse inversion imaging and related methods at very low MI allow real-time visualisation of perfusion using perfluorocarbon agents.

References

Apfel RE, HollandCK (1991) Gauging the likelihood of cavitation from short-pulse, low-duty cycle diagnostic ultrasound. Ultrasound Med and Biol 17:175-185

Becher H (1997) Second harmonic imaging with Levovist: initial clinical experience. In: Cate FT, deJong N (eds) Second European Symposium on Ultrasound Contrast Imaging. Book of Abstracts. Erasmus Univ, Rotterdam p 24

Becher H, Burns PN (2000) Handbook of Contrast echocardiography. Springer-Verlag Berlin, http://www.sunnybrook.utoronto.ca/EchoHandbook

Bleeker H, Shung K, Barnhart J (1990) On the application of ultrasonic contrast agents for blood flowmetry and assessment of cardiac perfusion. J Ultrasound Med 9:461-471

Brennan CE (1995) Cavitation and bubble dynamics. Oxford University Press, New York

Burns PN, Powers JE, Fritzsch T (1992) Harmonic imaging: a new imaging and Doppler method for contrast enhanced ultrasound. Radiology 185:142

Burns PN, Powers JE, Hope Simpson D, Uhlendorf V, Fritzsch T (1993) Harmonic contrast enhanced Doppler as a method for the elimination of clutter - In vivo duplex and color studies. Radiology 189:285

Burns PN, Powers JE, Hope Simpson D, Brezina A, Kolin A, Chin CT, Uhlendorf V, Fritzsch T (1994) Harmonic power mode Doppler using microbubble contrast agents: an improved method for small vessel flow imaging. Proc IEEE UFFC:1547-1550

Burns PN, Wilson SR, Muradali D, Powers JE, Fritzsch T (1996a) Intermittent US harmonic contrast enhanced imaging and Doppler improves sensitivity and longevity of small vessel detection. Radiology 201:159

Burns PN, Wilson SR, Muradali D, Powers JE, Greener Y (1996b) Microbubble destruction is the origin of harmonic signals from FS069. Radiology 201:158

Burns PN, Wilson SR, Hope Simpson D (2000) Pulse inversion imaging of liver blood flow: An improved method for characterization of focal masses with microbubble contrast. Invest Radiol 35:58-71

Child SZ, Hartman CL, Schery LA, Carstensen EL (1990) Lung damage from exposure to pulsed ultrasound. Ultrasound Med and Biol 16:817-825

Chin CT, Burns PN (1997) Predicting the acoustic response of a microbubble population for contrast imaging. In: Proc. IEEE Ultrason. Symp., pp 1557-1560

Dayton PA, Morgan KE, Klibanov AL, Brandenburger GH, Ferrara KW (1999) Optical and acoustical observations of the effects of ultrasound contrast agents. IEEE Transaction on Ultrasonics, Ferroelectrics, and Frequency Control 46:220-232

de Jong N (1997) Physics of microbubble scattering. In: Nanda NC, Schlief R, Goldberg BB (eds) Advances in echo imaging using contrast enhancement. Kluwer Academic Publishers, Dubai pp 39-64

Everbach EC, Makin IRS, Francis CW, Meltzer RS (1998) Effect of acoustic cavitation on platelets in the presence of an echo-contrast agent. Ultrasound Med and Biol 24:129-136

Hamilton MF, Blackstock DT (1998) Nonlinear acoustics. Academic Press, San Diego

Holland CK, Roy RA, Apfel RE, Crum LA (1992) In vitro detection of cavitation induced by a diagnostic ultrasound system. IEEE Trans. IEEE Transaction on Ultrasonics, Ferroelectrics, and Frequency Control 29:95-101

Hope Simpson D, Chin CT, Burns PN (1999) Pulse inversion doppler: a new method for detecting nonlinear echoes from microbubble contrast agents. IEEE Transactions UFFC 46:372-382

Kono Y, Moriyasu F, Nada T, Suginoshita Y, Matsumura T, Kobayashi K, Nakamura T, Chiba T (1997) Gray scale second harmonic imaging of the liver: a preliminary animal study. Ultrasound Med Biol 23(5):719-726

Miller DL, Gies RA, Chrisler WB (1997) Ultrasonically induced hemolysis at high cell and gas body concentrations in a thin-disk exposure chamber. Ultrasound Med and Biol 23:625-633

Miller DL, Thomas RM (1995) Ultrasound contrast agents nucleate inertial cavitation in vitro. Ultrasound Med Biol 21:1059-1065

Miller MW, Miller DL, Brayman A (1996) A review of in vitro bioeffects of inertial ultrasonic cavitation from a mechanistic perspective. Ultrasound Med and Biol 22:1131-1154

Mulvagh SL, Foley DA, Aeschbacher BC, Klarich KK, Seward JB (1996) Second harmonic imaging of an intravenously administered echocardiographic contrast agent: visualization of coronary arteries and measurement of coronary blood flow. J Am Coll of Cardiol 27:1519-1525

Neppiras EA, Nyborg WL, Miller PL (1983) Nonlinear behavior and stability of trapped micron-sized cylindrical gas bubbles in an ultrasound field. Ultrasonics 21:109-115

Ophir J, Parker KJ (1989) Contrast agents in diagnostic ultrasound [published erratum appears in Ultrasound Med Biol 1990;16(2):209]. Ultrasound Med Biol 15:319-333

Plesset MS (1949) The dynamics of cavitation bubbles. J Appl Mech 16:272-282

Poritsky H (1951) The collapse or growth of a spherical bubble or cavity in a viscous fluid. In: Sternberg E (ed) First U.S. National Congress on Applied Mechanics, Washington DC, pp 813-821

Porter TR, Xie F (1995) Transient myocardial contrast after initial exposure to diagnostic ultrasound pressures with minute doses of intravenously injected microbubbles. Demonstration and potential mechanisms. Circulation 92:2391-2395

Porter TR, Xie F, Kricsfeld D, Armbruster RW (1996) Improved myocardial contrast with second harmonic transient ultrasound response imaging in humans using intravenous perfluorocarbon-exposed sonicated dextrose albumin. Journal of the American College of Cardiology 27:1497-1501

Rayleigh L (1917) On the Pressure Developed in a Liquid During the Collapse of a Spherical Cavity. Philosophy Magazine Series 6:94-98

Taylor KJ, Burns PN, Wells PNT (1996) Clinical Applications of Doppler Ultrasound. New York: Raven Press

Tiemann K, Lohmeier S, Kuntz S, Koster J, Pohl C, Burns P, Porter TR, Nanda NC, Luderitz B, Becher H (1999) Real-time contrast echo assessment of myocardial perfusion at low emission power: first experimental and clinical results using power pulse inversion imaging. Echocardiography 16:799-809

Uhlendorf V, Hoffmann C (1994) Nonlinear acoustical response of coated microbubbles in diagnostic ultrasound. Proc IEEE Ultrasonics Symp:1559-1562

Uhlendorf V, Scholle F-D (1996) Imaging of spatial distribution and flow of microbubbles using nonlinear acoustic properties. Acoustical Imaging 22:233-238

Williams AR, Kubowicz G, Cramer E (1991) The effects of the microbubble suspension SHU 454 (Echovist) on ultrasound-induced cell lysis in a rotating tube exposure system. Echocardiography 8:423-433

Wilson SR, Burns PN (2001) Liver Mass Evaluation With Ultrasound: The impact of microbubble contrast agents and pulse inversion imaging. Sem in Liver Dis 21:147-161

Wilson SR, Burns PN, Muradali D, Wilson J, Lai X (2000) Harmonic Hepatic Ultrasound with Microbubble Contrast Agent: Initial experience showing improved characterization of hemangioma, hepatocellular carcinoma, and metastasis. Radiology 215:153-161

2 Ultrasound Contrast Agents

A. Bauer[†], L. Solbiati

2.1 Introduction

With the advent of new ultrasound contrast-specific scanning modes, the clinical potential of ultrasound contrast agents has been widely enhanced and the efficacy has been potentiated. Ultrasound contrast agents are based on microbubbles with a diameter of a few micrometers. Their efficacy was previously described mainly as echoenhancers for Doppler signals, and by enhancing the reflectivity of blood, the signal-to-noise ratio for Doppler signals can be enhanced and a clear Doppler trace may be obtained in otherwise difficult to scan patients.

With the new contrast-specific scanning modes, pulse sequences have been tailored to make use of the nonlinear properties of ultrasound contrast media; the signal from ultrasound contrast agent microbubbles is displayed as an image of the contrast agent microbubble distribution, similar to a digital subtraction angiography (DSA) image in X-ray angiography, separate from signals originating from tissue.

The role of ultrasound contrast agents is still changing, since today's clinical applications for ultrasound have developed over the years without the support of appropriate contrast agents.

In knowledge of the demand for precision and efficacy in medical diagnosis, the lack of contrast agents has left ultrasound in its infancy in many clinical applications.

X-ray and magnetic resonance (MR) contrast media are atomic in nature, the fundamental interaction leading to the efficacy of the contrast agent is a physical effect based on the use of atomic properties. The atoms leading to this effect are linked to molecules responsible for the favorable safety and pharmakokinetic properties of the contrast agents. In X-ray imaging, iodine atoms are the basis for increased radiodensity. In MR imaging, the paramagnetic properties of gadolinium are the basis for the imaging efficacy. X-ray and MR contrast media are usually very small, and therefore able to leave the vascular space by diffusion. Ultrasound contrast media, consisting of microbubbles, are relatively large entities. The size of the microbubbles, about 1-10 μm, is also the principal determinant of their physical efficacy. To be effective in the whole body, the microbubbles have to pass the lung capillaries after an i.v. injection. This imposes an upper limit on the size of the microbubbles, since larger microbubbles are readily exhaled in the lungs. The microbubbles surviving the lung filter are confined to the vascular bed, and cannot leak out to the extravascular space like X-ray or MR contrast agents since they are destroyed during this process of extravasation. Microbubbles are therefore true blood-pool contrast agents.

The clinical use of ultrasound contrast media started in the 1960s when Gramiak and Shah credited Claude Joyner with the observation of microbubble enhancement after the injection of indocyanine green into a cardiac catheter during M-mode scanning of the aortic valve (*Gramiak 1968*). Other dyes, saline, and even X-ray contrast media were all found to produce similar results, and it was soon recognized that the contrast effect was due to the presence of microbubbles. As the use of saline contrast became established in echocardiography, attempts were made to generate greater contrast by improving the microbubble yield. These attempts ranged from shaking the solution by hand prior to injection and varying the injection speed to the use of more elaborate devices consisting essentially of two syringes joined by a three-way stopcock, the agitated solution being obtained by repeatedly pumping the saline from one syringe to the other along with some air. In retrospect, most of these techniques can safely be described as rough and ready; however, they were only suitable for the production of very large microbubbles (>50 μm) whose size distribution was very poorly defined. It was not until 1984 that a method of producing smaller bubbles with a reasonably narrow size distribution was developed. Strong ultrasound fields have been used to generate microbubbles by means of sonication. The microbubbles in these sonicated preparations were of a size suitable for contrast (e.g., 8 ± 3 μm in 70 % dextrose). Their use was limited, however, as the microbubbles were unable to survive passage through the lungs after i.v. injection.

Since then, numerous attempts have been made to generate a reliable ultrasound contrast effect, most of which have been lacking reproducibility and consistency, mainly due to the difference in the bubble population and size distribution that results from variations of such preparations.

An interesting overview of these agitated solutions is given by Ophir and Parker (*Ophir 1989*).

2.2
Basic Physics and Pharmacology

Microbubbles provide the basis for all current developments in echocontrast media. The principal characteristic of microbubble-based ultrasound contrast media is their backscatter effect. When gas-filled microbubbles are present in a region of interest, a higher proportion of the ultrasound beam is backscattered and a stronger echo is received at the transducer than from the tissues alone and echogenicity is increased. The echogenicity of a medium, or degree of backscatter, is dependent on the medium's scattering strength. This can be expressed in terms of a parameter known as its scattering cross-section: an index of the efficiency of a scattering medium defined as the power scattered from a single source (bubble) divided by the intensity of the incident ultrasound ($\sigma = P/I$). Since the diameter of the microbubbles is small compared to the incident wavelength of the ultrasound field, the process is described as scattering, similar to the scattering of light by the molecules of the earth's atmosphere.

The underlying mechanism governing the scattering process is the difference in compressibility and density between the microbubbles' gaseous contents and the surrounding liquids. For a given microbubble, the number and size of microbubbles determine the intensity of the backscattered signal. Only a few microbubbles are needed to increase backscatter dramatically. A larger microbubble will result in a higher increase of the backscattered signal in off-resonance condition; however, the microbubble for diagnostic use has still to pass the capillary system of the lungs which impose the upper limit in the size of microbubbles.

Free, gas-filled microbubbles are very effective scatterers of ultrasound, but without some form of stabilization, they disintegrate rapidly and are unable to survive passage through the lungs after i.v. injection even if size requirements are met. To allow capillary passage, a thin shell sufficient to prevent diffusion of the gas - and, hence, disintegration of the bubbles - but with only a minimal effect on acoustic properties would be ideal. Attempts to produce coated microbubbles began as early as 1980 with the production of nitrogen filled-gelatin capsules. The size of the bubbles (about 80 μm) made them unsuitable for practical purposes, however. It was not until some time later that the technical difficulties in manufacturing reproducibly small microbubbles were finally solved.

The pharmacokinetics of echocontrast agents differs from that of X-ray or MR con-

Table 2.1. Transpulmonary ultrasound contrast media approved for clinical use

Ultrasound contrast media	Clinical indication
Albunex (Molecular Biosystems/Mallinckrodt)	LVO, not marketed
Optison (Molecular Biosystems/Mallinckrodt/Amersham)	LVO
Levovist (Schering)	Doppler enhancement
Sonovue (Bracco)	LVO, macrovascular and microvascular imaging
Definity (Bristol Myers Squibb)	LVO (USA and Canada), liver and kidney (Canada only)
Imagent (Alliance/Schering/Cardinal)	LVO (USA only)

LVO, Left Ventricular Output

trast media as they are not distributed throughout the body fluid but remain in the blood pool or in the body cavities to which they are applied. Therefore, the main areas of application are in echo enhancement of the blood flow in the heart chambers and blood vessels (blood pool contrast agents) and in the imaging of body cavities.

The short life-span of microbubbles in vivo is a fundamental problem. Pulmonary transit places high demands on bubble stability, and only very few preparations with the necessary bubble stabilization have reached the stage of clinical development. While the first generation of transpulmonary contrast agents used air as the gas in microbubbles (Albunex, Levovist), this resulted in short duration of the effect. The second generation of microbubble agents (SonoVue, Optison, Definity) uses rather insoluble gases such as SF6 or perfluorocarbons to achieve better stabilization of the microbubbles in vivo. With the second-generation ultrasound contrast media, the microbubbles are able to survive multiple capillary passages after an i.v. injection. This gives consistent echo enhancement in the left heart and the arterial system after i.v. injection as well as in the venous system after the second capillary passage (Table 2.1).

2.3
Commercial Ultrasound Contrast Media

The potential for echo-enhanced ultrasound was demonstrated experimentally at a relatively early stage, but it was only several years later,

that researchers were able to overcome all development problems and the first ultrasound contrast medium was finally approved for commercial distribution. Despite extensive effort and a variety of approaches, many interesting ultrasound contrast media are still in the phase of comprehensive testing and development.

2.3.1
Albunex™

Albunex™ (Molecular Biosystems, San Diego, CA, USA) was the first ultrasound contrast medium with transpulmonic properties to receive approval from a regulatory authority. The microbubbles in Albunex™ are enclosed in a coat of sonicated albumin. This provides the stabilization necessary for pulmonary transit. Albunex™ consists of three different protein fractions: a carrier fraction of 5% human serum albumin; an aqueous soluble fraction; and an aqueous insoluble fraction. It is supplied as a ready-to-use solution with a concentration of 300 to 500 $\times$ 10^6 microbubbles/ml. The mean diameter of the bubbles is about 4 µm, and 95 % are smaller than 10 µm. The plasma half-life is about 1 min (*Barnhart 1990*). Albunex™ has been approved for use in left and right heart studies in the USA, Japan and in some countries in Europe. It is no longer marketed since the availability of Optison, which uses the same technique with an optimized perfluor gas content.

2.3.2
Optison™

Optison™ (FSO 69) (Molecular Biosystems, San Diego, CA, USA) is a modification of Albunex™

with the same basic microbubbles coated with sonicated albumin. The gas enclosed in the microbubbles is perfluorpropane, a low-solubility perfluorcarbon gas that enhances microbubble stability after injection. The microbubbles are in the size range of 3.6–5.4 μm in diameter (*Dittrich 1995*). Clinically, Optison™ is superior to Albunex™, showing improved endocardial border definition with clinical conversion in 74% of 203 patients compared to 26% improved endocardial border definition with Albunex™ (*Cohen 1998*).

Optison™ is approved in both USA and Europe for enhancing the left ventricular border in cardiac imaging, and is currently distributed by Amersham (formerly marketed by Mallinckrodt).

2.3.3
Levovist®

Levovist® (SHU 508A, Schering AG, Berlin, Germany) is based on galactose microparticles as a vehicle for delivery of microbubbles of a defined size distribution. Its predecessor, Echovist®, uses the same basis for bubble formation; however, it lacks transpulmonary stability and is therefore limited to use for right heart contrast, assessment of right-to-left shunts and body cavities. Levovist® differs from Echovist® in that it contains palmitic acid, which acts as a surfactant and forms a thin coat around the microbubbles to achieve transpulmonary stability. Depending on the concentration used (200 mg/ml, 300 mg/ml, 400 mg/ml), signal enhancement of up to 25 dB is achieved with Levovist® (*Schwarz 1994*). The duration of enhancement is up to 5 min.

Levovist® is approved in Europe, Japan, Canada, and other countries for use in Doppler indications as a signal-enhancing agent in case of insufficient Doppler signal level at baseline.

2.3.4
SonoVue®

SonoVue® (BR1, Bracco, Milan, Italy) is a new echocontrast agent made of microbubbles stabilized by phospholipids and containing sulphur hexafluoride (SF6), an innocuous gas. The suspension shows a remarkable stability of more than 6 h after reconstitution, which allows preparation in advance without any practical hurdles.

The mean bubble diameter is 2.5 μm and more than 90% of the bubbles are smaller than 8 μm (*Schneider 1999*). SF6 enhances the resistance to pressure changes occuring in the left ventricle, in the pulmonary capillaries, or in the coronary circulation.

SonoVue® has proven its efficacy for Doppler enhancement in a wide variety of applications, such as transcranial and extracranial Doppler (*Bogdahn 1999*) as well as in arterial and venous enhancement of the body (*Leen 2002*) and in cardiac imaging (*Nanda 2002*).

SonoVue® has been successfully used with new techniques such as pulse inversion (*Solbiati 2001; Basilico 2002*) in liver imaging and has shown to be capable of imaging myocardial perfusion (*Agati 2002*).

SonoVue® is approved in Europe with a wide range of clinical applications including cardiac imaging, macrovascular and microvascular imaging. SonoVue NDA has been filed in the USA and is presently under evaluation by the FDA.

2.3.5
Definity™

Definity™ (ImaRx, Tucson, AZ, USA) (perflutren lipid microspheres) is based on microbubbles with lipid bilayers and octafluoropropane as stabilizing gas. The formulation was previously introduced with air and different gaseous contents as aerosomes (*Unger 1993*). It is already prepared in liquid form and is resuspended with a specially designed Vialmix™ apparatus. The resulting microbubbles are 1.1–3.3 μm in diameter with 98% less than 10 μm. The results of clinical trials in left ventricular imaging have shown improvement of endocardial border delineation in 91% of patients, with a mean duration of 90 s for the contrast effect (*Kitzman 2000*). Other indications are under development (*Rosenberg 2002*).

Definity™ is approved in the USA for improvement of delineation of the left ventricular border and is marketed by Bristol Myers Squibb (formerly marketed by DuPont). Definity is also approved in Canada for LVO, liver and kidney imaging.

2.3.6
Imagent™

Imagent™ (AFO 145, Alliance Pharmaceuticals, San Diego, CA, USA) is composed of surfactants, sodium chloride and phosphate buffers, presented as a dry powder in a vial that also contains gaseous perfluorohexane (*Pelura 1998*). The suspension is reconstituted with sterile water to give a preparation containing 90 µl/ml of perfluorohexane. The microbubble concentration is 5×10^8/ml and the mean bubble diameter is 6 µm.

Imagent™ was recently approved in the USA for improvement of delineation of the left ventricular border.

2.4
Future Developments in Ultrasound Contrast Media

Various avenues are being explored in the development of ultrasound contrast media, and a number of different substances with echocontrast potential have been presented in recent years.

New formulations of ultrasound contrast media have been using the stabilization of a hard shell rather than insoluble gases. Two formulations have been reported to be in clinical trials, SHU 563 (Schering) and Bispheres (Point Biomedical). This type of agent shows a remarkable stability and intense enhancement when used with high mechanical index scanning (*Bauer 1999*). Following i.v. administration and pulmonary transit, persistent enhancement is achieved even at very small doses. Using color Doppler, the particles can also be detected after enrichment in the reticuloendothelial system, above all in the liver. This provides a method of identifying tumor material by means of enhanced ultrasound. Since tumors do not contain any RES cells, selective enrichment of hard shell agents should enable their location in nonenhanced areas of the image. The development of organ-specific and function-specific agents for ultrasound diagnostics is an exciting area. However, the full benefits, possible applications, and particular advantages of individual preparations will only become apparent in the course of clinical testing over the next few years. Potentially, the incorporation of therapeutically effective drugs for local delivery will be the most prominent use for the hard shell microbubbles (*Dhond 2000*).

Recently it has been shown that other experimental agents can achieve a similar liver-specific late phase imaging even at low mechanical index scanning. BR 14 (Bracco), an agent under development, has shown this liver specific late phase, as has NC 100100 (Nycomed). The imaging of focal lesions in the delayed phase using specific microbubble properties will need further investigation regarding its clinical value.

In summary, today's progress in technology has led ultrasound contrast agents to a level of clinical utility and ease of use that has made them past of daily clinical practice. Current applications in Doppler enhancement and contrast-specific scanning show that this application will result in substantial changes of clinical practice and the position of ultrasound in the diagnostic arena will be reinforced by the use of ultrasound contrast media.

References

Agati L, Funaro S, Veneroso G, Volponi C, De Maio F, Madonna MP, Fedele F (2001) Non-invasive assessment of myocardial perfusion by intravenous contrast echocardiography: state of the art. Ital Heart J 2:403-437

Barnhart J, Levene H, Villapando E, et al (1990) Characteristics of Albunex, air-filled albumin microspheres for echocardiography. Invest Radiol 25:162-164

Basilico R, Blomley MJ, Harvey CJ, Filippone A, Heckemann RA, Eckersley RJ, Cosgrove DO. (2002) Which continuous US scanning mode is optimal for the detection of vascularity in liver lesions when enhanced with a second generation contrast agent? Eur J Radiol 41:184-191

Bauer A, Blomley M, Leen E, Cosgrove D, Schlief R (1999) Liver-specific imaging with SHU 563A: diagnostic potential of a new class of ultrasound contrast media. Eur Radiol 9 Suppl 3:S349-352

Bogdahn U, Holscher T, Rosin L, Gotz B, Schlachetzki F (1999) Contrast enhanced transcranial and extracranial duplex sonography: preliminary results of a multicenter phase II/III study with SonoVue-trade mark. Echocardiography 16:761-766

Cohen JL, Cheirif J, Segar DS (1998) Improved left ventricular endocardial border delineation and opacification with OPTISON (FS069), a new echocardiographic contrast agent. Results of a phase III Multicenter Trial. J Am Coll Cardiol 32:746-752

Dittrich HC, Bales GL, Kuvelas T (1995) Myocardial contrast echocardiography in experimental coronary artery occlusion with a new intravenously administered contrast agent. J Am Soc Echocardiogr 8:465-474

Dhond MR, Nguyen TT, Dolan C, Pulido G, Bommer WJ (2000) Ultrasound-enhanced thrombolysis at 20 kHz with air-filled and perfluorocarbon-filled contrast biospheres. J Am Soc Echocardiogr 13:1025-1029

Gramiak R, Shah PM (1968) Echocardiography of the aortic root. Invest Radiol 3:356-366

Kitzman DW, Goldman ME, Gillam LD, Cohen JL, Aurigemma GP, Gottdiener JS (2000) Efficacy and safety of the novel ultrasound contrast agent perflutren (Definity) in patients with suboptimal baseline left ventricular echocardiographic images. Am J Cardiol 86:669-674

Leen E, Angerson WJ, Yarmenitis S, Bongartz G, Blomley M, Del Maschio A, Summaria V, Maresca G, Pezzoli C, Llull JB (2002) Multi-centre clinical study evaluating the efficacy of SonoVue (BR1), a new ultrasound contrast agent in Doppler investigation of focal hepatic lesions. Eur J Radiol 41:200-206

Nanda NC, Wistran DC, Karlsberg RP, Hack TC, Smith WB, Foley DA, Picard MH, Cotter B (2002) Multicenter evaluation of SonoVue for improved endocardial border delineation. Echocardiography 19:27-36

Ophir J, Parker KJ (1989) Contrast agents in diagnostic ultrasound. Ultrasound Med Biol 15:319-333

Pelura TJ (1998) Clinical experience with AF0150 (Imagent US), a new ultrasound contrast agent. Acad Radiol 5 [Suppl 1]:S69-71

Rosenberg ML, Carpenter AP (2002) Contrast material-enhanced abdominal US examinations with DMP 115 (DEFINITY) provides additional diagnostic information with potential for changes in patient management. Acad Radiol 9 [Suppl 1]:S243-245

Schneider M (1999) Characteristics of SonoVue. Echocardiography 16:743-746

Schwarz KQ, Becher H, Schimpfky C, Vorwerk D, Bogdahn U, Schlief R (1994) A Study of the magnitude of Doppler enhancement with SH U 508 A in multiple vascular regions. Radiology 193:195-201

Solbiati L, Tonolini M, Cova L, Goldberg SN (2001) The role of contrast-enhanced ultrasound in the detection of focal liver leasions. Eur Radiol 11 [Suppl 3]:E15-26

Unger E, Shen DK, Fritz T, Lund P, Wu GL, Kulik B, DeYoung D, Standen J, Ovitt T, Matsunaga T (1993) Gas-filled liposomes as echocardiographic contrast agents in rabbits with myocardial infarcts. Invest Radiol 28:1155-1159

3 Liver Physiology

D. BECKER

3.1 Introduction

The liver is a unique organ having a dual role as a metabolic and biochemical transformation factory. The liver receives blood containing substances absorbed or secreted by the unpaired gastrointestinal organs. These substances are raw materials and the liver modifies them and synthesizes new chemicals which are then returned to the bloodstream or to bile for excretion.

On a cellular level, liver cells are organized into cell plates, each plate being formed by one-cell-thick cords, which are surrounded by blood vessels (so-called sinusoids). The perfusion of these sinusoids is unidirectional from the portal branch to the hepatic venule. The specialized capillaries found in these sinusoids normally have (in liver healthy persons) large fenstrations which allow exchange between plasma and the extracellular space.

First, the basic elements of the organization of the liver will be described, thereafter the anatomic organization of the liver will be explained with the gross anatomy of the liver, biliary system, and the blood vessels supplying both venous and arterial blood to the liver. Later, the structure of the liver lobule will be discussed, including a description of the nonparenchymal cells: endothelial cells, Kupffer cells, stellate cells, and pit cells. These nonparenchymal cells contribute to normal liver function in various important roles both in health and following hepatic injury. Lastly, the functional organization of the cell plate will be described with emphasis on the uptake of compounds from plasma into hepatocytes, their metabolism and biotransformation.

3.2 Anatomy

The liver is the largest gland in the human body and accounts for approximately 2.5% of total body weight. In the adult, the liver weighs almost 1,500 g. The liver is divided into four lobes. Although one might think that the left and right lobe are seperated in the patient's middle line, they are in fact separated by the falciform ligament. Thus, part of the left lobe is located at the patient's right side. These lobes are supplied by the right and left branches of the portal vein and the hepatic artery. Bile is drained from the liver by the left and right hepatic ducts. The right and the left lobes can be further divided into segments according to the surgical anatomy of Couinaud (Figs. 3.1, 3.2). This segmentation of the liver arises from the possibility of surgical resection of each segment due to the vessel anatomy.

The falciform ligament separates as it proceeds superiorly. There is, therefore, a segment on the superior surface of the liver that is not covered with peritoneum. This is the so-called *bare area* (area nuda in Latin). Besides this peritoneal covering, the entire liver is covered by a thin connective tissue capsule (Glisson's capsule). This capsule completely surrounds the liver and consists of collagen fibers with accompanying small blood vessels. The capsule is thickest near the porta hepatis and the

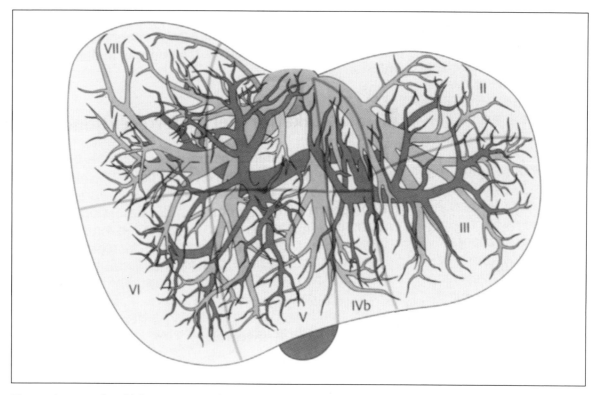

Fig 3.1. Segmental and lobar anatomy of the liver according to Couinaud. The braches of the hepatic veins are shown in *light gray*, those of the portal vein in *dark gray* (adapted from *Koeckerling 2000*). The *roman numbers* represent the liver segments

inferior vena cava.

The blood supply to the liver is unique because it has a dual source. Under physiologic conditions the portal vein carries the majority (75%) of the afferent blood volume to the liver. The remaining 25% is supplied by blood from the hepatic artery (*Kruger et al. 2000*). These two vessels, along with their accompanying connective tissue, enter the liver through the porta hepatis. The porta hepatis is the area where the blood vessels enter and bile duct leaves the liver. It is contained in folds of the hepatoduodenal ligament. The vessels quickly arborize into smaller branches and ultimately form the blood channels of the liver sinusoids.

Under physiologic conditions (after a fasting period), the liver is perfused with 1,500 ml blood per minute, during portal venous and arterial blood flow as described above. The total amount of blood flow changes after a meal and can also change during rest or when the liver undergoes various diseases. This means that during rest, approximately 30% of the car-

diac output flows into and through the liver.

In patients with liver cirrhosis, the cardiac ouput is often increased leading to a larger amount of blood passing the liver during rest. Due to portal hypertension, the amount of arterial blood flow is increased and the portal venous flow is decreased. This can be measured using Doppler sonography (*Kruger et al. 2000*). It is not yet clear if this change in blood flow shows a correlation with the severity of liver damage and if this can be used to monitor the progress of liver fibrosis. Currently this is under investigation (*Albrecht et al. 1999; Bernatik et al. 2002a*).

Another condition where there is a change in blood flow is the occurrence of liver metastases. These metastases often have exclusive arterial blood supply. This leads to a shift in the relationship between arterial and portal blood flow, increasing the arterial part. These conditions can also be measured using Doppler ultrasound and, perhaps, the transit time of echo-enhancing agents in (or through) the liver.

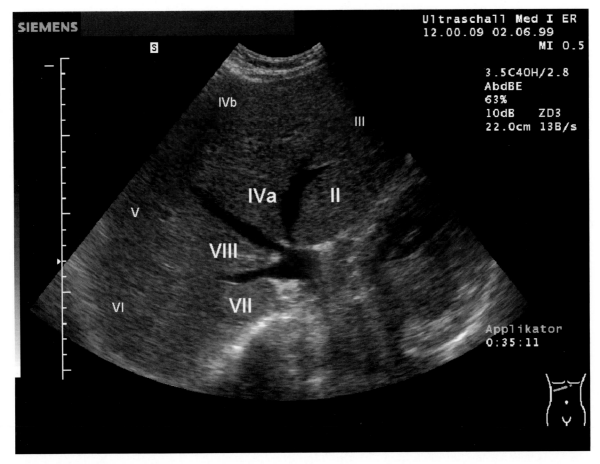

Fig. 3.2. Sonographic view of the lobar anatomy according to Couinaud's segments, subcostal view. *Roman numbers* represent liver segments

Whether this tool is useful for the detecion of small liver metastases is also currently under investigation (*Bernatik et al. 2002b*).

The gallbladder serves as a reservoir for bile. It is located on the undersurface of the right lobe. In healthy humans, it may hold 30–50 ml of bile when fully distended. In its contracted state it has numerous rugae similar to those found in the stomach. Layers of smooth muscle form an elastic muscularis. The serosal surface consists of numerous collagen fibers, blood vessels, and lymphatics as well as nerves from the autonomic nervous system.

The neck of the gallbladder terminates in the cystic bile duct. A series of folds form the "spiral valves." The cystic duct joins the common hepatic duct and forms the common bile duct. As the common bile duct passes through the duodenal wall it is surrounded by the sphincter of Oddi. The components of the sphincter of Oddi regulate flow of bile and pancreatic enzymes into the duodenum.

3.3
Liver Lobule Structure

3.3.1
Liver Cell Plate

Histologic units within the liver parenchyma have been reported since the late 1600s. Most modern textbooks of histology provide detailed descriptions of two primary models of organization of the liver lobule. These are the classic lobule and the liver acinus. These two models describe the identical hepatic structure and are only different interpretations of hepatic organization. The classic lobule contains liver tissue with boundaries made by connective

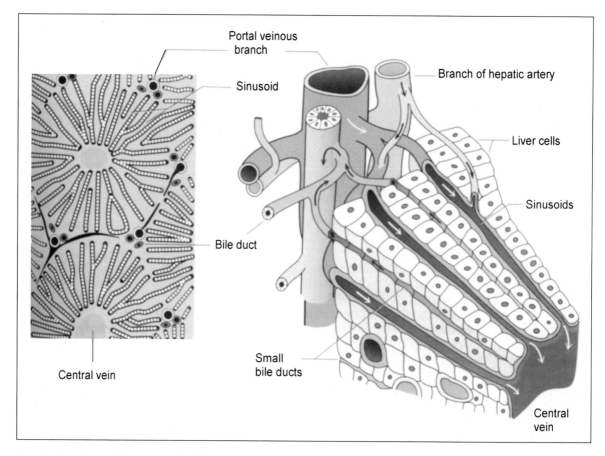

Fig. 3.3. Lobular architecture of the liver. (Adapted from *Gebhardt 2000*)

tissue. These are most prominent in nonhuman species such as the pig. The typical appearance is that of a hexagon with portal triads at the corners of the hexagon. In the center of the hexagon is the central vein. The liver cell plates radiate from the central vein to the portal triads, which are located at the circumference of the lobule. The lobulation in humans appears less well defined with no sharp demarcation between lobules owing to a paucity of connective tissue (Fig. 3.3).

In the pioneering work of Rappaport, the organizational unit of the human liver was defined as an acinus. In this model, three concentric zones surround the portal triad. The cells close to the hepatic veins are most likely to be damaged by ischemia.

Blood enters the liver sinusoid through the portal tract via the portal vein and hepatic arteriole. Blood from these vessels empties into the hepatic sinusoids and flows unidirectionally along the liver cell plate. As it exits the cell

plate, it empties into the central vein. Bile flows in the opposite direction to the blood thus forming a countercurrent system similar to that in the kidney.

3.3.2
Nonparenchymal Liver Cells

The liver contains various different cells of distinct function. Classically, liver cells are divided into parenchymal cells (hepatocytes) and nonparenchymal cells. These cell types have various functions. This group of nonparenchymal cells includes endothelial cells, Kupffer cells, hepatic stellate cells, and pit cells.

3.3.3
Sinusoidal Endothelial Cells

For the liver to function as a major metabolic factory there must be rapid and full exchange between the blood and liver cell. This requires special features within the sinusoidal endothelium to ensure such permeability. In addition to allowing rapid exchange of both large and small molecules between sinusoidal plasma and the hepatocyte surface, sinusoidal endothelial cells have an important filtration role. The endothelial cell, when seen on electron microscopy, has a flattened profile. Rather than forming a continuous boundary, small gaps are found in the cell cytoplasm. These gaps, known as fenestrae, occur in patches and allow proteins to move freely from the sinusoidal plasma into the space of Disse. The space of Disse varies in size and contains microvilli from hepatocytes that protrude into the sinusoidal lumen through the fenestrae.

Marked changes occur in the sinusoidal endothelial cells in response to liver injury, for example, fibrosis or cirrhosis. All of these yield reduced endothelial permeability. The most striking feature is that the number of fenestrae decreases. In addition, a real continuous basal membrane forms beneath the endothelium. The space of Disse becomes filled with collagen bundles, thus further reducing the access of solutes to liver cells. This so-called capillarization of sinusoids has functional implications that have been documented using multiple indicator dilution curves in cirrhotic human and rat livers. This change in sinusoidal permeability leads to impaired liver clearance of solutes and seems to be irreversible. Hopefully we will be able to use this capillarization as a diagnostic tool to monitor the progression of fibrosis in patients with chronic liver diseases [(see Chapter 3.2, Anatomy (*Albrecht 2000; Bernatik 2002a*)].

3.3.4
Kupffer Cells

Kupffer cells are liver macrophages that were first described by Kupffer in 1876. They are currently described as cells that have phagocytic activity and are located along the lining of the sinusoid. Kupffer cells are difficult to identify by light microscopy alone, and proper identification depends on using immunohisto- chemical techniques. Research techniques involving phagocytosis of latex particles have been used to identify Kupffer cells. Therefore, the cytoplasm of Kupffer cells often contains cellular debris intermixed with degradative lysosomes.

Kupffer cells account for 2.1% of the nonparenchymal cells on a volume basis. The origin of these cells in the liver has remained controversial. Two current theories are that Kupffer cells are derived from circulating monocytes or by local self-perpetuation. Studies using human liver transplantation samples have demonstrated that the Kupffer cell population acquires the genotype of the recipient several months after transplantation. This observation would suggest that Kupffer cells come from circulating monocytes. Other studies using mouse macrophages have demonstrated that Kupffer cells are generated from promonocyte-like precursors.

Whatever the source of Kupffer cells, it is clear that they are markedly decreased in cirrhosis. It has been speculated that cirrhosis causes portosystemic shunting of cytokines, decreasing the Kupffer cell population. The loss of Kupffer cells may lead to the increased susceptibility to infections in cirrhosis due to bacteria in the portal vein.

Kupffer cells, like hepatic stellate cells and macrophages in the other parts of the body, undergo activation. Under the influence of numerous biologic mediators, they become stimulated and continue their phagocytic role. When stimulated, they secrete numerous products, including cytokines, fibronectin, prostaglandins, platelet activating factor, and transforming growth factor (TGF)-β.

In addition to clearing bacteria from portal blood, Kupffer cells also remove viruses during viremia. During viral hepatitis in humans, Kupffer cells undergo hyperplasia. Each of the hepatitis viruses has been identified in Kupffer cells during chronic hepatitis as well as acute infection; it is unclear whether the cleared viruses are actually destroyed. In this situation, Kupffer cells may serve as a reservoir for the virus, thus extending the period of viremia.

Finally, Kupffer cells are the primary site of endotoxin removal. Endotoxin circulates systemically during sepsis caused by gram-negative bacteria. Initial studies suggested that Kupffer cell uptake of endotoxin was beneficial. However, recent studies have suggested that endotoxin-mediated Kupffer cell release of tumor necrosis factor (TNF)-α may contribute to a lethal shock of sepsis.

3.3.5
Hepatic Stellate Cells

The biology of hepatic stellate cells has become the topic of intense investigation. However, the knowledge of the existence of the cells dates to 1876 when Kupffer identified these cells using a gold chloride histochemical technique. Confusion about their phagocytic capabilities continued to exist in the literature until 1951 when Ito suggested that hepatic stellate cells and Kupffer cells (as we now know them) were separate cell populations. Hepatic stellate cells are now known to represent a discrete population of nonparenchymal cells. Their most characteristic feature is that their cytoplasm contains large amounts of retinoids. They can be identified by the natural fluorescence of these vitamin A-like compounds.

Despite comprising only about a third of the nonparenchymal cells, hepatic stellate cells are recognized to play an important role in fibrogenesis in various liver diseases. The unique morphology and ultrastructure of hepatic stellate cells have allowed their identification. In normal liver, they are located primarily in the periportal region of sinusoids closely approximating the endothelial cells. Hepatic stellate cells have been shown to be contractile, and it has been proposed that they could regulate sinusoidal blood both in normal or injured liver.

3.3.6
Fibrosis and Hepatic Stellate Cells

Literature data suggest that hepatic stellate cells, like other nonparenchymal cells, may undergo "activation" when the liver is injured. For hepatic stellate cells, this "activation" involves the transition from a resting cell to one that is predominantly a protein-secreting cell. During this activation, the hepatic stellate cell loses its vitamin A stores, develops receptors to various cytokines and proteins, and begins to secrete type I collagen. While they are activated, hepatic stellate cells express several smooth muscle markers.

Recent research has demonstrated that hepatic stellate cells are the major producers of the collagen found in cirrhosis. While the resting stellate cell produces small amounts of collagen types III and IV, the activated cell produces primarily collagen type I but also collagen III, IV, VI, fibronectin, hyaluronic acid, and other proteins. This matrix deposition by hepatic stellate cells seems to occur regardless of the type of liver injury and has been documented in human illnesses including viral and alcoholic hepatitis and hemochromatosis.

In addition to vitamin A storage and matrix protein synthesis, hepatic stellate cells perform several other roles in humans. They express erythropoietin, hepatocyte growth factor, colony-stimulating factor, and epidermal growth factor. The role that hepatic stellate cells play in the biology of these compounds is an area of current research. Finally, recent studies have demonstrated that hepatic stellate cells may function in the regulation of blood flow to sinusoids. Hepatic stellate cells undergo contraction when stimulated by several mediators and may regulate blood flow to individual sinusoids as well as causing whole organ shunting in cirrhosis.

3.3.7
Pit Cells

Pit cells are the most recently recognized group of cells of the nonparenchymal cell types. They are also known as natural killer (NK) cells. They are generally found within the sinusoidal lumen and are rare cells, being only about 20 % as numerous as Kupffer cells. Their name is attributable to the first description by Wisse, when they were noted to have dense granules in their cytoplasm that resembled pits. In contrast to Kupffer cells, pit cells are nonphagocytic and do not have any endogenous peroxidase activity. Their identification relies on characteristic antigens that they express. All pit cells express OX-8 antigens just as NK cells do. However, unlike NK cells in the blood, pit cells do not express the T cell antigen OX-19. Knowledge of the function of pit cells is rapidly emerging. Current evidence suggests that pit cells are part of the liver's antitumor defense. This is based on studies in which pit cells were observed to lyse lymphoma cells and cancer cells in culture, in the absence of other cells such as Kupffer cells. There exists a large body of experimental evidence using both human and animal cell lines which suggests that NK cells provide an important barrier in tumor defense. Recent evidence has also documented the accumulation of pit cells in viral hepatitis in humans. It is unclear whether pit cells are able to destroy virus-infected hepatocytes. Current thinking suggests that they may play a role both in the clearance of hepatotropic viruses as well as in tissue rejection after orthotopic liver transplantation.

3.4
Hepatocyte Transport

3.4.1
Electrolyte and Solute Transport

One of the principal functions of the liver is bile formation. There is a great deal of information regarding the mechanism by which individual hepatocytes extract electrolytes and solutes from the plasma, transport them across the plasma membrane, and excrete them into bile. Numerous transport mechanisms are associated with the sinusoidal plasma membrane. Specific transporters have been identified to facilitate the uptake of hydrophilic bile acids, amino acids, and organic anions such as sulfobromophthalein. All of these transporters rely on the potential difference maintained across the hepatocyte membrane (-35 mV) and the inward sodium concentration gradient.

Bile acids also enter hepatocytes by specific transporters located on the sinusoidal plasma membrane. Most studies have supported a sodium-coupled transporter for most of the bile acids found in humans. The hydrophobic unconjugated bile acids are transported more efficiently than are conjugated trihydroxy bile acids. This suggests that some bile acids may partition into the lipid bilayer without the need for a specific energy-dependent pump.

3.4.2
Bile Formation

The purpose of bile formation by the liver is twofold: bile formation represents an important route of excretion for substances that have been extracted from plasma, metabolically altered by the liver and excreted into bile. Bilirubin is a classic example. The second major function of bile is to aid in the absorption of lipids and fat-soluble substances. The bile acids are uniquely suited for this function.

Bile formation begins with hepatocytes actively secreting bile acids and electrolytes. Inorganic solutes including bilirubin and various hydrophobic drugs are also excreted into bile. Current evidence suggests that water follows by passive diffusion maintaining the isoosmotic status with plasma. In the bile ducts, canalicular bile is further modified with secretion of water and electrolytes. During storage in the gallbladder, electrolytes are reabsorbed. The exact contribution of secretion and the absorption by the canalicular cells is unclear, owing to the technical difficulty of measuring the chemical composition of bile in the canaliculi.

3.5
Functional Organization of the Liver Cell Plate

The organisation of liver tissue centers around the individual liver cell plate. The cell plate is formed along a single sinusoid by a layer of hepatocytes, one cell thick and comprises 15–20 hepatocytes (Fig. 3.3). The plate extends from the portal space to the hepatic venule. Because each hepatocyte is approximately 30 µm across, the average length of a cell plate is approximately 500 µm. In addition to the hepatocytes, nonparenchymal cells also line the sinusoids.

In this section, liver function that is performed within the liver cell plate is discussed, concentrating on the design of the liver cell plate and how it affects hepatic function. Several features make this design unique. The unidirectional flow of plasma along the liver cell plate allows functional compartmentation to develop. Because of this, cells exposed to blood near the portal inlet are in contact with the highest concentration of incoming solutes including oxygen. These cells are primarily responsible for the uptake of toxic compounds, whereas cells farther downstream are more active in the secretion of metabolic byproducts. Thus, as the plasma flows from its portal inlet to its hepatic outlet, its composition is modified. This leads to a dramatic difference in the microenvironment surrounding each hepatocyte and leads to a variety of injury patterns that are well documented in clinical practice.

3.5.1
Limiting Plate

The limiting plate is defined as the row of hepatocytes that surrounds the portal space. It is from this location in the liver cell plate that bile leaves the hepatocytes that formed it. Bile moves along the liver cell plate in bile canaliculi and moves in a countercurrent direction compared with blood flow. Scanning electron microscopy has shown that bile canaliculi are approximately 1 µm in diameter. As they leave the liver cell plate, the bile canaliculi form bile ductules (canals of Hering). The bile ductules are formed by cuboidal cells which form a duct that is 1–3 µm in diameter. As these canaliculi combine, they form an ampulla that is located at the junction of the limiting plate and the portal space. Bile flow along the bile ductule is enhanced by biliary cilia (7–15 µm) which run in the direction of bile flow. The bile ductules then form bile ducts as the bile leaves the limiting plate and proceeds into the biliary system.

3.5.2
Hepatocyte Heterogeneity Along the Liver Cell Plate

Along the liver cell plate, hepatocytes in general appear histologically uniform. However, when examined on a morphologic or histochemical basis, hepatocytes exhibit marked heterogenicity. This heterogenicity (also called zonation) is manifested by cells located in the periportal zone that differ from those downstream in the perivenous zone. Hepatocytes

demonstrate zonation with respect to key enzymes, cell receptors, subcellular structures and cell matrix interaction. The heterogenicity is expressed by activation of the cellular genome in response to various inputs, including concentration gradients in hormones, oxygen, metabolic substrates, and neural input.

In the 1960s und 1970s, it became clear that there was a zonal organization for specific groups of enzymes and the concept of "metabolic zonation" became popular. In the orignal model of metabolic zonation, only two zones of equal size were defined. Later as the concept of zonation became more popular, the periportal and perivenous compartments were subdivided into a proximal and distal part creating four zones.

3.5.3
Carbohydrate Metabolism

Zonation of carbohydrate metabolism is divided into two phases: absorptive and postabsorptive. During the absorptive phase, glucose is primarily taken up by the perivenous cells. In these cells, it is used to synthesize glycogen. Following replacement of glycogen stores, glucose is converted to lactic acid and released into the hepatic veins. Lactic acid is then taken up by the periportal cells, where it is used as a substrate for gluconeogenesis. This concept is consistent with the observation that glycogen stores are refilled first in the perivenous hepatocytes whereas glycogen degradation starts periportally.

In the postabsorptive phase, glycogen is degraded to glucose in the periportal hepatocytes. As the glucose proceeds down the sinusoid it is taken up by perivenous cells and degraded to lactate. Lactate is again released into the circulation and, if unused by the peripheral circulation, it is used as a substrate for gluconeogenesis by periportal cells.

3.5.4
Fatty Acid Metabolism

The zonation of fatty acid metabolism is less pronounced than that described for carbohydrate metabolism. Perivenous cells appear to synthesize preferentially very low-density lipoprotein whereas periportal cells perform β-oxidation and ketogenesis. Fatty acid-binding protein, the chief intracellular transport protein for long-chain fatty acids, is located predominantly in periportal cells. It is unclear whether the presence of this intracellular carrier promotes the preferential β-oxidation and ketogenesis seen in periportal cells. 3-Hydroxy-3-methylglutaryl coenzyme A (HMG-CoA) reductase is located almost exclusively in periportal cells.

3.5.5
Amino Acid and Ammonia Metabolism

Nutrient proteins in the form of amino acids are supplied to hepatocytes via the portal vein. Periportal cells preferentially convert the NH3 to urea. If the quantity of ammonia presented to the periportal region is sufficient to escape ureagenesis, perivenous hepatocytes take up the NH3 and convert it to glutamine. Glutamine is then released into the systemic circulation and returned to periportal cells, where again the NH3 is preferentially formed into urea. The periportal and perivenous systems have different kinetics with the periportal system being a high-capacity, low-affinity pathway and the perivenous pathway having a high affinity but a low capacity. Studies using perfused livers have demonstrated that the removal of ammonia in periportal cells (urea synthesis) is restricted to incoming ammonia concentrations higher than 50 μm and that glutamine synthesis in the perivenous cells occurs at concentrations of ammonia below 50 μM.

3.5.6
Regulation of Hepatocyte Heterogenicity

It is generally assumed that hepatocyte zonation develops as a consequence of the heterogenicity in the microenvironment of individual cells. This is controlled by various signals such as substrate concentration (including oxygen), hormones, neuromediators, nerves, and cell-to-biomatrix interactions. The differential expression patterns seen in the zonation may be attributed to different rates of mRNA transcription, mRNA degradation, mRNA translation, or end-protein degradation.

The expression of the genes for the enzymes of gluconeogenesis is regulated at the pretranslational level. Similarly, the amino acid metabolizing enzymes are regulated at the pretransitional level. Each of these alterations in gene expression occurs during a normal feeding rhythm. In contrast, glycolytic enzymes appear to be regulated mainly at the post-translational level during a normal feeding pattern. Each of these generalities regarding the regulation of zonal gene expression may change depending on the nutritional conditions.

Ammonia detoxification also appears to be regulated at the pretranslational level. Both the mRNA and the proteins of the key ureagenic enzymes are located exclusively in the periportal cells. In contrast, the mRNA and the protein for glutamine synthesis are located exclusively in parenchymal cells in the distal perivenous area. Neither these mRNAs nor the enzyme levels themselves seem to vary with the nutritional state, suggesting that the organism needs to maintain tight control over ammonia despite external influences.

3.5.7
Physiologic Significance of Hepatocyte Heterogenicity

The pattern of organization described earlier indicates the complexity of the liver's ability to respond to a large variety of input and output solute concentrations and the overmetabolic demands of the organism. Two control elements seem to dictate the degree of zonal responses: the sequent delivery of substrates and the zonal patterns of gene expression. Because of the unidirectional perfusion of the liver acinus, periportal cells are exposed to a high concentration of incoming solutes. Solutes using transport systems that have a great capacity for uptake (NH3 and bile acids) are preferentially taken up by the first hepatocytes that they encounter. Refluxed material or substances escaping uptake in periportal cells are subsequently presented to "downstream cells." The removal of ammonia, either as urea or by glutamine synthesis, is an example of this complex control system. Each of these systems allows minute adjustments to the outflow concentration of substances of a splanchnic organ as well as new products formed by the synthetic machinery of the liver.

In summary, the zonation of hepatocytes allows the liver acinus to accomplish the regulation of substrate production and the metabolism of proteins and hormones in a dynamic fashion. Zonation appears to depend on the unidirectional perfusion of substrates as well as on basic gene expression by hepatocytes. Each of these control mechanisms is dynamic, responding to the overall needs of the organism.

References

Albrecht T, Blomley MJ, Cosgrove DO, Taylor-Robinson SD, Jayaram V, Eckersley R et al (1999) Non-invasive diagnosis of hepatic cirrhosis by transit-time analysis of an ultrasound contrast agent. Lancet 353:1579-83

Bernatik T, Strobel D, Hahn EG, Becker D (2002a) Doppler measurements: a surrogate marker of liver fibrosis? Eur J Gastroenterol Hepatol 14:383-387

Bernatik T, Strobel D, Hausler J, Wein A, Hahn EG, Becker D (2002b) Hepatic transit time of an ultrasound echo enhancer indicating the presence of liver metastases - First clinical results. Ultraschall Med 23:91-95

Gebhardt R (2000) Funktionen der Leber und ihre Regulation. In: Hahn EG, Riemann JF (eds) Klinische Gastroenterologie Vol. 3. Thieme, Stuttgart New York, pp 1437-1462

Koeckerling F (2000) Funktionelle Anatomie der Leber. In: Hahn EG, Riemann JF (eds) Klinische Gastroenterologie Vol. 3. Thieme, Stuttgart New York, pp 1430-1436

Kruger S, Strobel D, Wehler M, Wein A, Hahn EG, Becker D (2000). Hepatic Doppler perfusion index - a sensitive tool for detection of liver metastases? Ultraschall Med 21:206-209

4 Macro- and Microcirculation of Focal Liver Lesions

4.1
Traumatic Abdominal Lesions

A. MARTEGANI, L. AIANI

4.1.1
Introduction

Ultrasound (US) plays a secondary role to computed tomography (CT) in the diagnostic assessment of traumatic lesions involving abdominal organs, especially in the case of major trauma (*Becker et al. 1998; Boioli et al. 1993; Brown et al. 1998; Harris et al. 2001; Mirvis 2000; Sherck et al. 1984; Shuman 1997*). Because US has a relatively limited panoramic capacity, it does not detect lesions of hollow internal organs reliably. On the whole it has a lower sensitivity and specificity than CT in the diagnosis of parenchymal damage to the liver, kidney and spleen.

We must also bear in mind the drawback that US depends heavily on the skill of the operator and that in this type of pathology we need a rapid diagnosis..

Nonetheless, US has two important advantages over CT: its portability, which means that it can be done virtually anywhere, and its repeatability.

Moreover, we should consider that in grading the severity of trauma, there are mild abdominal trauma conditions which in practice demand only clinical monitoring (with laboratory tests at most). For these cases, US serves as a stand alone imaging procedure (*Richardson et al. 1997; Brown et al. 2001; Dulchavsky et al. 2002; Freeman 1999; Kirkpatrick et al. 1997: Lenz et al. 1996; Lingawi and Buckeley 2000; McGahan et al. 1999; Porter et al. 1997; Weill et al. 1998*).

It is in this context that we include our preliminary experience using contrast-enhanced ultrasound (CEUS) in traumatic abdominal pathologies (*Basilico et al. 2002; Burns et al. 1996, 2000; Del Favero et al. 2000; Mattrey and Pelura 1997*).

4.1.2
Ultrasound and Abdominal Trauma

Currently, the main reason for using US is to detect effusions, primarily intraperitoneal effusions. This diagnostic goal can be easily and rapidly achieved and provides the basis for so-called FAST ultrasound (Fig. 4.1).

US suffers from the drawbacks mentioned above in the detection of traumatic parenchymal lesions, especially in the acute phase. Using a contrast medium, however, can make it far easier to recognize parenchymal lesions – as shown in the following image gallery.

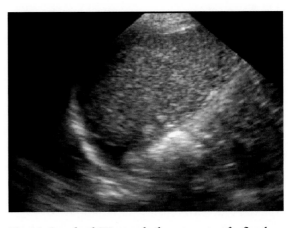

Fig 4.1. Standard US reveals the presence of a fine layer of perisplenic fluid effusion

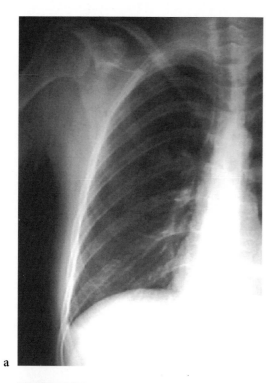

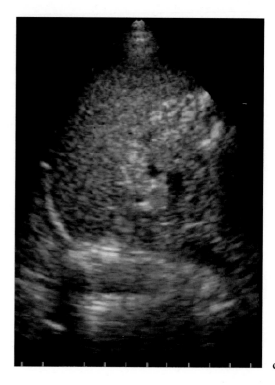

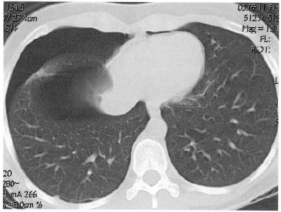

Fig 4.2 a-c. Case 1. **a** Chest X-ray: small area of right margino costal PNX. **b** Chest CT: confirms the PNX with a small area of lung contusion. **c** Standard US: no evidence of focal splenic lesions

4.1.3
Contrast-Enhanced Ultrasound Image Gallery

CASE 1

Clinical history: A 28 year-old road accident victim with no apparent consequences apart from mild trauma of the right chest (Fig. 4.2).
Chest X-ray: Small area of right pneumothorax (PNX) with no rib fractures.
Normal blood chemistry parameters.
No particular subjective symptoms.

Diagnosis: Intraligament rupture of the splenic parenchyma.
Comment: This was a case of minor trauma with no apparent damage to the peritoneal organs. Both CT and standard US revealed a very fine perihepatic effusion.
CEUS detected a transcapsular lesion of the spleen and correctly identified the diffusion path of the hematoma. It is worth noting that the CEUS examination of the spleen can be done at the end of the hepatorenal assessment (up to 4–5 min after injecting the contrast medium) if a conservative low mechanical index (MI) technique is used.

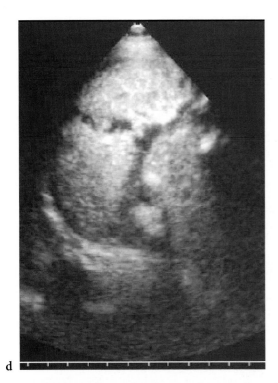

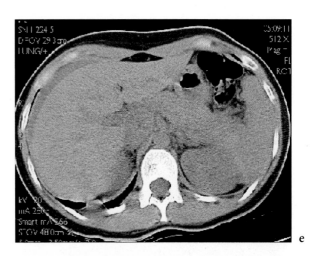

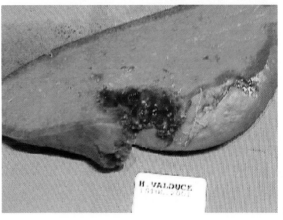

Fig 4.2 d-f. Case 1. **d** CEUS: 60 s after injection of the contrast medium. Full-thickness lesion with hypoechogenic collection at pancreatic-splenic ligament level. **e** Standard CT: hyperdense appearance due to recent hemorrhage at pancreatic-splenic ligament level, heterogeneous structure of the spleen. **f** Detail of the surgical specimen

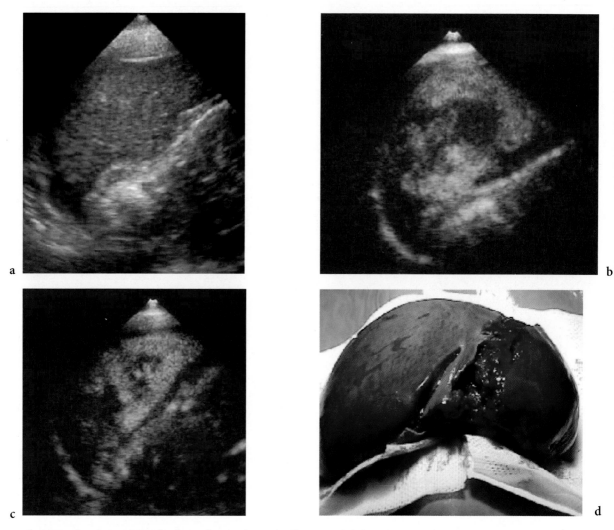

Fig. 4.3 a-d. a Case 2. Standard US: free peritoneal effusion in left hypochondrium with hyperechogenic hetero-geneity of the spleen. **b-c** CEUS: rupture of the splenic parenchyma with subcapsular hematoma and free perisplenic effusion. **d** Surgical specimen confirming the splenic rupture

CASE 2

Patient examined directly at the emergency room (Fig. 4.3).
Clinical history: Road accident victim with no apparent vertebra or rib fractures. Stationary clinical conditions (no shock) but severe ab-dominal pain on the left side accompanied by pallor. Mild anemia.
Diagnosis: Splenic lesion with rupture of the capsule and hemoperitoneum
Comment: CEUS was performed less than 2 min after injecting the contrast agent and did not prolong the examination time significantly. The splenic origin of the hemoperitoneum was

easily identified. Moreover, CEUS showed the extent and topography of the effusions more clearly than standard US.

CASE 3

Clinical history: Unremarkable domestic acci-dent involving a patient with chronic pancre-atitis known to have moderate splenomegaly (Fig. 4.4).
Comment: Splenectomy revealed a lesion of the splenic parenchyma with no laceration of the capsule. No signs of active bleeding were iden-tified. In this case, the CEUS did not demon-strate active bleeding.

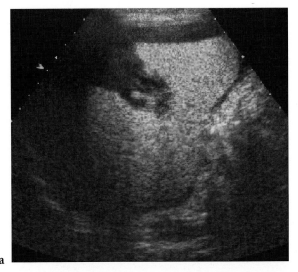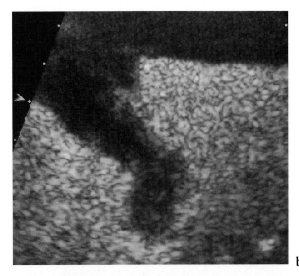

a   b

Fig. 4.4 a,b. a Case 3. CEUS: splenic lesion and severe perisplenic hematoma. No diffuse hemoperitoneum. **b** Detail of CEUS revealing the absence of microbubbles outside the damaged splenic parenchyma

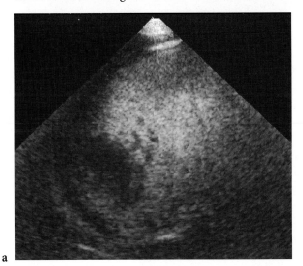

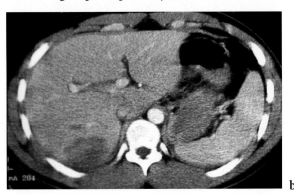

b

Fig. 4.5 a,b. a Case 4. CT (done when the patient was admitted to the intensive care unit): area of hepatic contusion with no evidence of perihepatic bleeding. **b** CEUS (obtained at the bedside 24 h later): showing the area of contusion and a small perihepatic fluid effusion

a

CASE 4

Patient hospitalized in intensive care (Fig. 4.5).
Clinical history: Road accident.
CT of the brain, chest and abdomen performed.
A hepatic contusion with no significant hemoperitoneum had been diagnosed.
Diagnosis: Hepatic contusion.
Comment: CEUS allows an easy and close monitoring of hepatic parenchymal lesions. The search for traumatic lesions can be done during the portal phase, 60 sec after injecting the contrast agent, and protracted for 1–2 minutes. In this case, CEUS identified a small perihepat-

ic hemorrhage which was easily controlled on a daily basis without any particular harm to the patient.

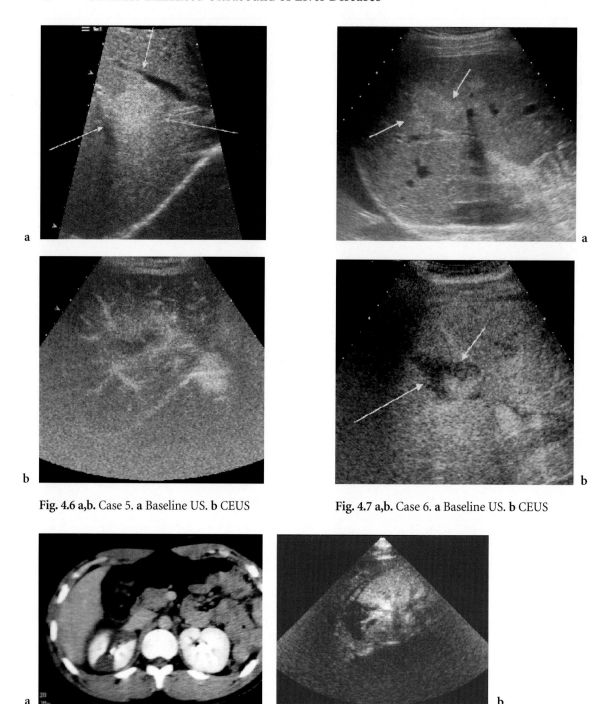

Fig. 4.6 a,b. Case 5. **a** Baseline US. **b** CEUS   **Fig. 4.7 a,b.** Case 6. **a** Baseline US. **b** CEUS

Fig. 4.8 a,b. Case 7. **a** Contrast-enhanced CT: demonstrates a localized avascular appearance of the right kidney with no perirenal effusion of contrast medium and with a very fine layer of hepatorenal fluid effusion. **b** CEUS: avascular appearance of the superior renal pole with no avulsion of the collector system, which is still in its normal position

CASES 5 and 6

Case 5: Sport trauma (fall from bicycle) with blunt abdominal trauma. Patient stable (Fig. 4.6).
Case 6: Sport trauma with blunt abdominal trauma (Fig. 4.7).

Comment: In both cases, CEUS showed an avascular area that appeared on standard US as a hyperechogenic hepatic contusion. With CEUS, the margins and therefore size were easier to identify.

CASE 7

Clinical history: Contusion and pain on the right side due to a sport trauma. Asymptomatic patient (Fig. 4.8).

Comment: To identify lesions clearly, the kidneys must be studied within 2 min of contrast administration. Given the relatively rapid fading of the contrast medium, the investigation of each kidney must be performed separately.

4.1.4
Conclusions

CEUS has several advantages over standard US for monitoring patients with blunt abdominal traumas, in terms of the immediate recognition of the image corresponding to the lesion and the speed of examination. Moreover, CEUS can be repeated as often as needed and has no side effects.

Although our limited experience does not allow us to reach any final conclusions, the prospects for clinical use of CEUS seem to be good, especially for studying the spleen.

References

Basilico R, Blomley MJ, Harvey CJ, et al (2002): Which continuous US scanning mode is optimal for the detection of vascularity in liver lesions when enhanced with a second generation contrast agent? Eur J Radiol 41:184-191

Becker CD, Mentha G, Terrier F (1998): Blunt abdominal trauma in adults: role of CT in the diagnosis of visceral injuries. Part 1: liver and spleen. Eur Radiol 8:553-562

Boioli F, Gattoni F, Tagliaferri B, et al (1993): Role of computed tomography in splenic blunt trauma. Radiol Med 85:213-217

Brown M, Casola G, Sirlin CB (2001) Blunt abdominal trauma: screening US in 2693 patients. Radiology 218:352-358

Brown SL, Hoffman DM, Spirnak JP (1998) Limitations of routine spiral computerized tomography in the evaluation of blunt renal trauma. J Urol 160:1979-1981

Burns PN, Powers JE, Simpson DH, et al. (1996) Harmonic imaging with ultrasound contrast agents Clin Radiol 51 [Suppl 1]:50-55

Burns PN, Wilson SR, MD, Simpson DH (2000) Pulse inversion imaging of liver blood flow: improved method for characterizing focal masses with microbubble contrast. Invest Radiol 35:58-71

Del Favero C, Martegani A, Aiani L, et al Liver imaging: to break or not to break the microbubbles? Syllabus Bubbles in Radiology - the State of the Art. The Second Symposium on Ultrasound Contrast for Radiological Diagnosis 44-51; Oct 22-23 2000, Toronto, Canada

Dulchavsky SA, Henry SE, Moed BR, et al (2002) Advanced ultrasonic diagnosis of extremity trauma: the FASTER examination. J Trauma 53:28-32

Freeman P (1999) The role of ultrasound in the assessment of the trauma patient Aust J Rural Health 7:85-89

Harris AC , Zwirewich CV, Liburn ID, et al (2001) CT findings in blunt renal trauma. Radiographics 21:201-214

Kirkpatrick AW, Simons RK, Brown R, et al (2002) The hand-held FAST: experience with hand-held trauma sonography in a level-I urban trauma center. Injury 33:303-308

Krupnick AS, Teitelbaum DH, Geiger JD, et al (1997) Use of abdominal sonography to assess pediatric splenic trauma. Potential pitfalls. Ann Surg 225:408-414

Lenz KA, McKenney MG, Numez DB Jr, et al (1996) Evaluating blunt abdominal trauma: role for ultrasonography. J Ultrasound Med 15:447-451

Lingawi SS, Buckeley AR (2000) Focused abdominal US in patients with trauma Radiology 217:426-429

Mattrey RF, Pelura TJ (1997) Perfluorocarbon-based ultrasound contrast agents. In: Goldberg BB (ed) Ultrasound contrast agens. Martin Dunits, pp 83-87

McGahan JP, Richards JR, Jones CD, et al (1999) Use of ultrasonography in patients with acute renal trauma. J Ultrasound Med 18(3):207-213

Mirvis SE (2000) Role of CT in diagnosis and management of spleen injury. Appl Radiol 29:7-12

Porter RS, Nester BA, Dalsey WC, et al (1997) Use of ultrasound to determine need for laparotomy in trauma patients. Ann Emerg Med 29:323-330

Richardson MC, Hollman AS, Davis CF (1997) Comparison of computed tomography and ultrasonographic imaging in the assessment of blunt abdominal trauma in children. Br J Surg; 84:1144-1146

Sherck JP, McCort JJ, Oakes DD (1984) Computed tomography in thoracoabdominal trauma. J Trauma 24:1015-1021

Shuman WP (1997) CT of blunt abdominal trauma in adults. Radiology 205:297-306

Weill F, Rohmer P, Didiel D, et al (1988) Ultrasound of the traumatized spleen; left butterfly sign in lesions masked by echogenic blood clots. Gastrointestinal Radiol 13:169-172

4.2
Hepatic Hemangiomas

A. Martegani, C. Borghi

4.2.1
Anatomical and Structural Features

Hemangioma is the most common focal lesion of the liver, with an incidence in the general population that ranges from 7% to 20% (based on autopsy findings).

Although it occurs more frequently in females, it is not particularly prevalent in any given age bracket.

The finding of multiple hemangiomas is frequent, often associated with multiple cysts, in a picture of diffuse or organ-specific multiple angiomatosis (Rendu-Osler-Weber disease).

From an anatomopathological point of view, hemangioma can be divided into two main types:

• Capillary hemangioma
• Cavernous hemangioma.

Capillary hemangiomas are relatively small (<3 cm) and have very fine vascular structures. Some types of capillary hemangiomas, usually those smaller than 2 cm, may have highly concentrated arterial microvessels (high-flow hemangiomas). Generally, however, their appearance is mixed, characterized by the presence of nodules with peripheral arterial vascularization and venous lakes.

Cavernous hemangiomas usually are larger (>3 cm) and combine fine vascular branches with ample venous lakes. Giant forms of hemangioma (>10 cm) can also occur. Although hemangiomas have no capsule, cavernous hemangiomas may show a non homogeneous structure with venous lakes alternating with areas composed of dense connective tissue or thrombosed portions.

Neither type shows any arterial-venous microfistulas. Inflow is due mainly, but not exclusively, to a tributary from the hepatic artery; portal inflow is absent or negligible.

Macro-vascular structures, with a diameter greater than 200 microns, are virtually never detected inside a hemangioma. Entirely thrombosed forms are extremely rare. The single vessels present a wall comprising a single endothelial layer.

From a topographical standpoint, hemangiomas are more common in the right lobe of the liver. They occur more frequently in the region under the Glissonian capsule or along the main intrahepatic vessels, especially the suprahepatic veins. In this case, if small, hemangiomas characteristically do not include any dislocation or infiltration of the affected vein.

4.2.2
Diagnostic Imaging

Hemangiomas are best detected with ultrasound. They are usually found incidentally since, except for the relatively rare giant angiomas, the vast marjority are asymptomatic (*Gandolfi et al. 1991; Marn et al. 1991; Mirk et al. 1982; Moody and Wilson 1993; Onodera et al. 1983*).

Capillary hemangiomas usually appear as small lesions (<3 cm) that are hyperechogenic with respect to the surrounding parenchyma (except in the case of markedly steatotic infiltrations). They have smooth, distinct margins and a homogeneous structure (Fig. 4.9).

Cavernous hemangiomas are more likely to have larger lesions with heterogeneous structure and variable echogenic response, along with frankly hypoechogenic areas coinciding with the venous lakes (Fig. 4.10).

The lesion margins are clear; pseudo-capsular features are rare and are always due to vascular structure displacement by the larger lesions. Although posterior echo enhancement can be detected in cavernous hemangiomas, it is more common in the capillary type.

Ultrasound cannot be considered specific in all cases. Given their structural diversity, cavernous hemangiomas must be differentiated from primary and secondary liver neoplasms. In capillary hemangiomas, it is important to consider the differential diagnosis with respect to hyperechogenic metastases (neuroendocrine tumors) and, in the case of patients with cirrhosis, to hyperplastic nodules or genuine hepatocellular carcinoma.

Color-Doppler or power-Doppler may suggest a benign diagnosis by demonstrating the absence of vascular signals inside the lesion. In

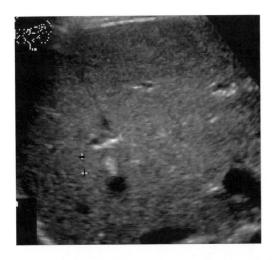

Fig 4.9. Small capillary angioma with the typical appearance of a hyperechogenic, well-defined lesion

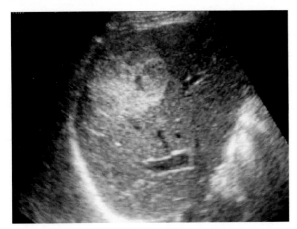

Fig 4.10. Heterogeneous appearance of a paravasal cavernous angioma

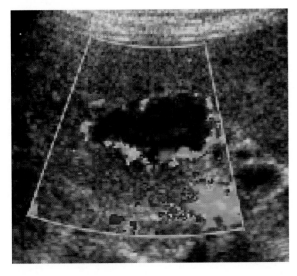

Fig 4.11. Abundant perivasal circulation surrounding a capillary angioma

fact, hemangiomas may reveal vessels that can only be sampled at the periphery of the lesion (Fig. 4.11) (*Tanaka et al. 1987*).

Sporadic intralesional flows may be identified in the case of high-flow hemangiomas and capillary hemangiomas. It is important to note that the absence of intralesional flows is by no means rare, even in small or amply necrotic neoplastic lesions.

4.2.3
Integrated Imaging

Given the above considerations, integrated imaging of hemangiomas is commonly used to improve specificity.

The methods most frequently used are computed tomography (CT) and magnetic resonance imaging (MRI), while nuclear medicine and angiography are rarely used (*Freeny and Marks 1986; Heiken et al. 1989; Jang et al. 1998; Unal et al. 2002; Yun et al. 1999; Van Beers et al. 1997; Van Leuwen et al. 1996*).

Contrast-enhanced CT scanning can diagnose hemangiomas with sequential scans that demonstrate the progressive centripetal filling of the lesion after the intravenous administration of a contrast agent (Fig. 4.12).

MRI allows the same dynamic assessment, but is also capable of identifying the characteristic hyperintensity of the signal in the long TR and TE sequences, which reflects the abundant free water content (Fig. 4.13).

4.2.4
Contrast-Enhanced Ultrasound Imaging

The use of a conservative technique, causing little or no contrast medium microbubble destruction during insonation at low mechanical index (MI), together with a second generation contrast agent, allows monitoring of the angio-dynamic behavior of a hemangioma, the specific features of which are usually sufficient to diagnose its nature (*Basilico et al. 2002; Burns et al. 1996, 2000; Del Favero et al. 2000; Jang et al. 2000; Kim et al. 2000 a, b; Leen 2001; Leen et al. 2002; Lee et al. 2002; Quaia et al. 2002; Wilson et al. 2000*).

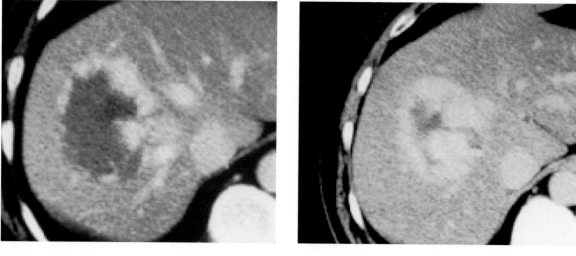

Fig. 4.12 a,b. Progressive centripetal impregnation of a cavernous angioma demonstrated at dynamic CT in the portal and late phases

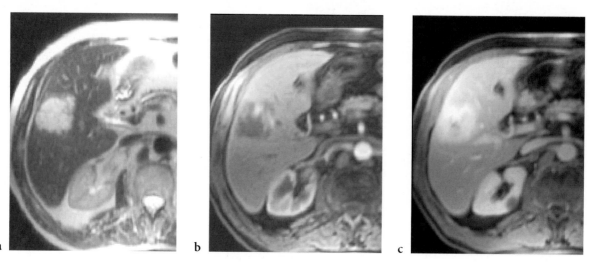

Fig. 4.13 a-c. a Typical T2-dependent hyperintensity of the angiomatous lesion. **b** Lively impregnation at the periphery of the angioma in the arterial phase (20 s). **c** Centripetal enhancement in the late phase (3 min).

Essentially there are three vascular phases to consider:

1. Arterial inflow phase (approximately 20 s after the injection of the contrast medium)
2. Portal inflow phase (from 60 to 240 s after the injection of the contrast medium)
3. Late phase (4-5 minutes after the injection of the contrast medium)

In the arterial phase, both capillary and cavernous hemangiomas, usually demonstrate an early, strong peripheral enhancement. This enhancement may have a globular appearance (Fig. 4.14) or show signs of ring of various thickness and uniformity (Fig. 4.15).

To be considered as an exception are high-flow hemangiomas, that show strong, early generalized enhancement as well as the rare finding of completely thrombosed or fibrosed hemangioma, which reveals a total lack of arterial inflow (Fig. 4.16).

In the portal phase, hemangioma shows a tendency for centripetal filling that may be complete (Fig. 4.17) or incomplete (Fig. 4.18).

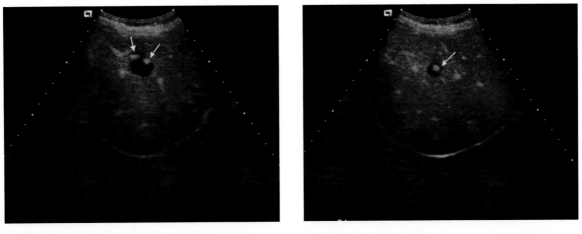

Fig. 4.14 a,b. Peripheral enhancement with large globules visible in the arterial phase

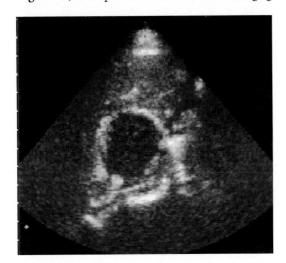

Fig. 4.15. Variability of enhancement peripheral to continuous swelling

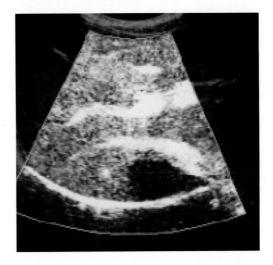

Fig. 4.16. Total absence of impregnation in the late arterial phase (40 s) in a case of completely thrombosed angioma

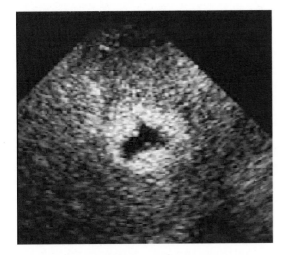

Fig. 4.17. Example of incomplete impregnation of the central portion in the late phase (3 min)

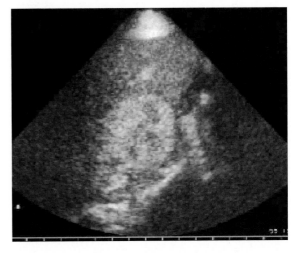

Fig. 4.18. Complete impregnation with angioma totally hyperechogenic 3 minutes after injecting the contrast agent

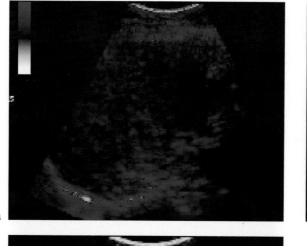
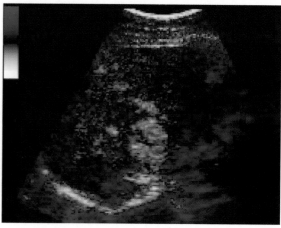
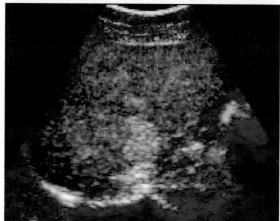

Fig. 4.19 a–c. a Baseline image. **b** Strong impregnation (enhancement) of high-flow angioma in the arterial phase. **c** The lesion is hyperechogenic in the late phase (4 min)

In high-flow hemangioma, the echogenicity of the lesion – reflecting its degree of vascularization – tends to be much the same as the surrounding parenchyma (Fig. 4.19) or slightly hyperechogenic.

In the case of thrombosed hemangiomas, the signs of hypovascularization – and consequently of hypoechogenicity – remain the same.

In the late phase, the vascular components of both capillary (Fig. 4.20) and cavernous (Fig. 4.21) hemangiomas tend to appear relatively hyperechogenic in comparison with the surrounding hepatic parenchyma.

Due to incomplete filling of the lesion, a certain degree of structural diversity is more common in cavernous hemangiomas.

In the case of thrombosed hemangiomas, the avascular (and hypo-anechogenic) appearance persists (Fig. 4.22).

Further confirmation can be obtained by su-

perimposing B mode on low MI color mode imaging. This can simultaneously demonstrate the microvascular enhancement of the lesion and the absence of intralesional macrovessels, which is quite common (Fig. 4.23).

Characterization of the hemangioma is based on the following flow characteristics:

- Peripheral arterial inflow
- Slow centripetal enhancement
- Late uptake of microbubbles

4.2.5
Differential Diagnostic Problems

Metastases often show peripheral arterial inflow but generally do not have a tendency for centripetal diffusion. Moreover, they present a rapid outflow and are consistently hypoechogenic in the late phase.

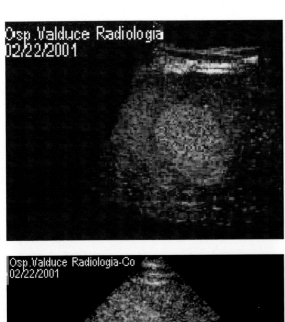

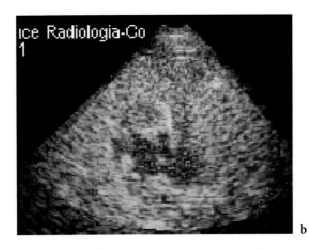

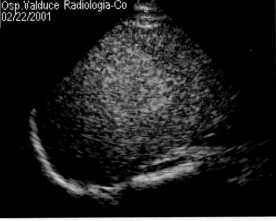

Fig. 4.20 a-c. a Baseline: capillary angioma. **b** Impregnation is still incomplete in the portal phase. **c** The lesion remains hyperechogenic in the late phase (4 min).

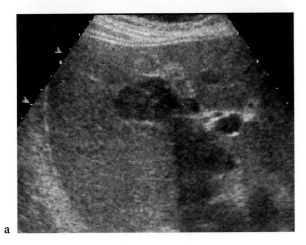

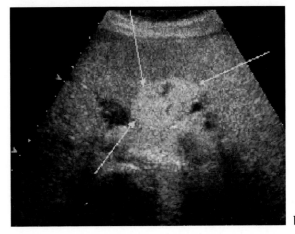

Fig. 4.21 a,b. a Baseline: cavernous angioma. **b** The lesion is hyperechogenic, but not completely opaque, in the late phase

In addition, an arterial inflow (central or peripheral) is always detectable, even in the case of hypovascular metastases while it is not observed in thrombosed hemangiomas.

Unlike hepatocellular carcinomas, high-flow hemangiomas are impregnated also in the late phase, revealing a hyperechogenic appearance generally stronger than is seen in focal nodular hyperplasia.

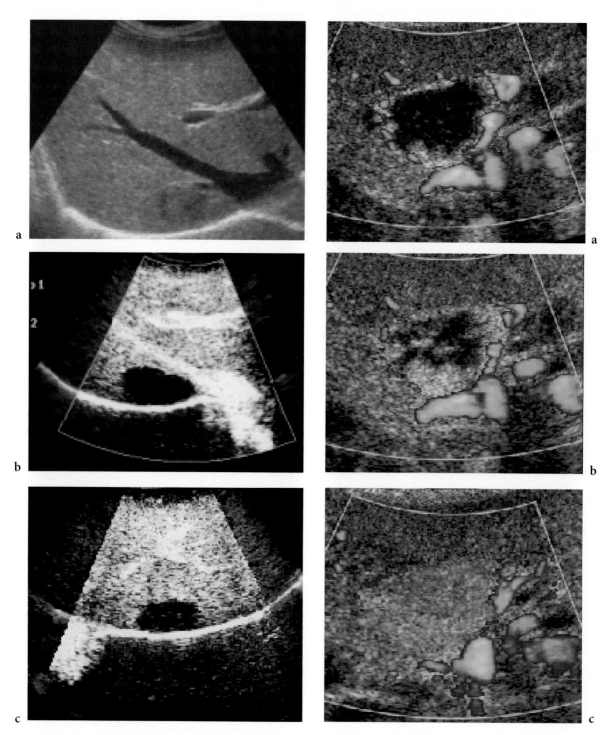

Fig. 4.22 a-c. a Baseline: thrombosed angioma. **b** Late arterial phase. **c** Late phase: the lesion is constantly hypoechogenic and avascular

Fig. 4.23 a-c. Progressive impregnation demonstrated by the increment in the echogenicity of the lesion on the gray scale. Macrovessels are clearly evident at the periphery of the lesion, but are never detectable inside the lesion

References

Basilico R, Blomley MJ, Harvey CJ, Filippone A, Heckemann RA, Eckersley RJ, Cosgrove DO (2002). Which continuous US scanning mode is optimal for the detection of vascularity in liver lesions when enhanced with a second generation contrast agent? Eur J Radiol 41:184-91

Burns PN, Powers JE, Simpson DH, et al (1996) Harmonic imaging with ultrasound contrast agents Clin Radiol 51 [Suppl 1]:50-55

Burns PN ,Wilson SR, MD, Simpson DH (2000) Pulse inversion imaging of liver blood flow: improved method for characterizing focal masses with microbubble contrast. Invest Radiol 35:58-71

Del Favero C, Martegani A, Aiani L, et al (2000) Liver imaging: to break or not to break the microbubbles? Syllabus Bubbles in radiology - the state of the art. The Second Symposium on Ultrasound Contrast for Radiological Diagnosis, Toronto, Canada, pp 44-51

Freeny PC, Marks WM (1986) Hepatic hemangioma: dynamic bolus CT. AJR Am J Roentgenol 147:711-19

Gandolfi L, Leo P, Solmi L et al (1991) Natural history of hepatic hemangiomas: clinical and ultrasound study. Gut 32:677

Heiken JP, Weyman PJ, Lee JKT et al (1989) Detection of focal hepatic masses: prospective evaluation with CT, delayed CT, CT during arterial portography and MRI. Radiology 171:47-52

Jang HJ, Choi BI, Kim TK et al (1998) Atypical small hemangiomas of the liver: "bright dot" sign at two-phase spiral CT. Radiology 208:543-548

Jang HJ, Lim HK, Lee WJ et al. (2000) Ultrasonographic evaluation of focal hepatic lesions: comparison of pulse inversion harmonic and conventional imaging techiniques. J Ultrasound Med 19(5):293-299; quiz 301-302

Kim KW, Kim TK, Han JK et al (2000) Hepatic hemangiomas: spectrum of US appearances on gray-scale, power Doppler, and contrast-enhanced US. Korean J Radiol 1:191-197

Kim TK, Choi BI, Han JK et al, (2000) Hepatic tumors: contrast agent enhancement patterns with pulse inversion harmonic US. Radiology 216, 411-417

Marm MA, Bree RL, Siver TM (1991) Ultrasonography of the liver: technique and focal and diffuse disease. Radiol Clin N Am 29:1151

Mirk P, Rubaltelli L, Bazzocchi M, et al (1982) Ultrasonographic patterns in hepatic hemangiomas. J Clin Ultrasound 10:373-378

Moody AR, Wilson SR (1993) Atypical hepatic hemangioma: a suggestive sonographic morphology. Radiology 188:413-417

Onodera H, Ohta K, Oikawa M, et al (1983) Correlation of the real-time ultrasonographic appearance of hepatic hemangiomas with angiography. J Clin Ultrasound 11:421-425

Tanaka S, Kitamura T, Fuijta M et al (1987) Color Doppler flow imaging of liver tumors. AJR 154:509

Unal O, Sakarya ME, Arslan H et al (2002) Hepatic cavernous hemangiomas: patterns of contrast enhancement on MR fluoroscopy imaging. Clin Imaging 26:39-42

Van Beers BE, Gallez B, Pringot J (1997) Contrast-enhanced MR imaging of the liver. Radiology 203:297-306

Van Leeuwen MS, Noordzij J, Feldberg MAM, et al (1996) Focal liver lesions: characterization with triphasic spiral CT. Radiology 201:327-36

Yun EJ, Choi BI, Han JK, et al (1999) Hepatic hemangioma: contrast-enhancement pattern during the arterial and portal venous phases of spiral CT. Abdom Imaging 24:262-266

Lee JY, Choi BI, Han JK, et al (2002) Improved sonographic imaging of hepatic hemangioma with contrast-enhanced coded harmonic angiography: comparison with MR imaging. Ultrasound Med Biol 28(3):287-95

Leen E (2001) The role of contrast-enhanced ultrasound in the characterisation of focal liver lesions. Eur Radiol 11 [Suppl 3]:E27-34

Leen E, Angerson WJ, Yarmenitis S, (2002) et al Multicentre clinical study evaluating the efficacy of SonoVue (BR1), a new ultrasound contrast agent, in Doppler investigation of focal hepatic lesions. Eur J Radiol 41:200-206

Quaia E, Bertolotto M, Dalla Palma L, (2002) Characterization of liver hemangiomas with pulse inversion harmonic imaging. Eur Radiol 12:537-544

Wilson SR, Burns PN, Muradali D, et al (2000) Harmonic hepatic US with microbubble contrast agent: initial experience showing improved characterization of hemangioma, hepatocellular carcinoma and metastasis. Radiology 215 (1):153-161

4.3
Hepatic Adenoma

L. SOLBIATI, M. TONOLINI, A. BELLOBUONO

Hepatic adenoma (HA) is an uncommon primary benign tumor of hepatocellular origin. Most cases occur in young females and are related to the use of hormonal medications. Oral contraceptives and androgen steroid therapy have been recognized as causative agents and their withdrawal may result in regression of the lesion. Patients affected with type-I glycogen storage disease are at high risk of developing adenomas (*Ros 2001*).

Adenoma may be an asymptomatic incidental finding or may present with pain due to mass effect. Differentiation of adenoma from other benign or malignant liver masses, such as focal nodular hyperplasia (FNH), conventional or fibrolamellar hepatocellular carcinoma or hypervascular metastasis may be difficult. However, correct diagnosis and treatment of HA is clinically relevant because this tumor has a marked tendency to intralesional or life-threatening intraperitoneal bleeding and a potential – although very rare – for malignant transformation.

HA is a solitary (in 80% of cases), well-circumscribed and often encapsulated tumor. It owes its characteristic hypervascular behavior to large subcapsular feeding vessels originating from the hepatic arterial system. Histolog-ically it is composed of cords of proliferating hepatocytes, usually containing significant amounts of glycogen and fat, among which bile ductules, portal venous tracts and terminal hepatic veins are absent (*Ros 2001*). Intralesional calcifications and fibrosis are very rare. Excess growth in respect to its vascular supply explains the appearance of hemorrhagic and necrotic changes in large lesions.

Liver adenomatosis is a rare entity which is diagnosed in patients without a history of metabolic disease or steroid medication presenting with multiple adenomas, usually affecting both lobes. The histopathologic and imaging features of these lesions are not specific, but the disease tends to be progressive and symptomatic leading to hemorrhage, impaired liver function and sometimes malignant degeneration (*Grazioli 2000*).

The sonographic appearance of HAs is variable and nonspecific: most commonly it is a well-defined nodule or mass, according to its size. The high lipid content of hepatocytes may result in variable to uniform hyperechogenicity within the lesion (Fig. 4.24a). Bleeding usually leads to internal inhomogeneity, with hyperechoic areas in lesions with acute bleeding, and/or hypo- to anechoic areas corresponding to older hemorrhages.

Color Doppler may assist in the correct diagnosis, demonstrating large peripheral subcapsular arteries and veins and intratumoral venous vessels (*Golli 1994*).

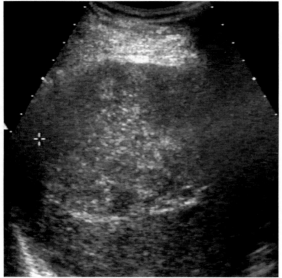

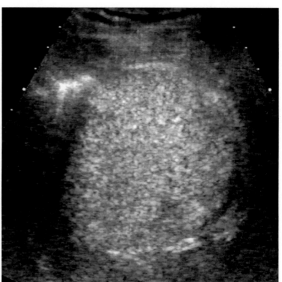

a

b

→

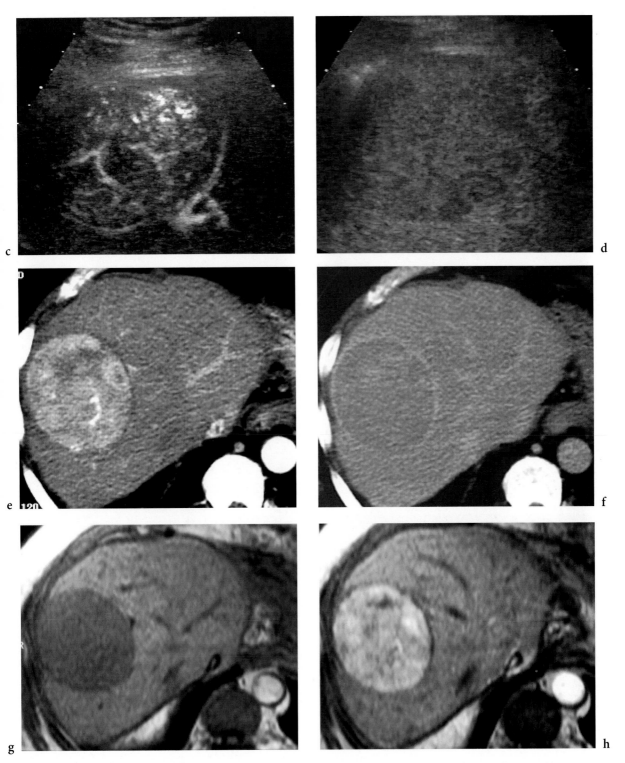

Fig. 4.24 a-g. Large (7.5 cm) hepatic adenoma at segment 8. **a** On baseline US, predominantly hyperechoic mass with peripheral hypoechoic rim. **b** On low-MI CEUS, in arterial phase (15-20 s after contrast administration), the mass enhances homogeneously. Increasing MI (to 0.40) the parenchymal microvasculature of the mass is significantly less well depicted, while pericapsular feeding arteries are clearly seen (**c**). In portal phase the washout of the adenoma occurs faster than that of the surrounding liver, with the mass appearing slightly hypoechoic (**d**). Similar findings are achieved with contrast-enhanced CT in arterial (**e**) and portal phases (**f**), and baseline T1-weighted (**g**) and gadolinium-enhanced T1-weighted (**h**) MRI

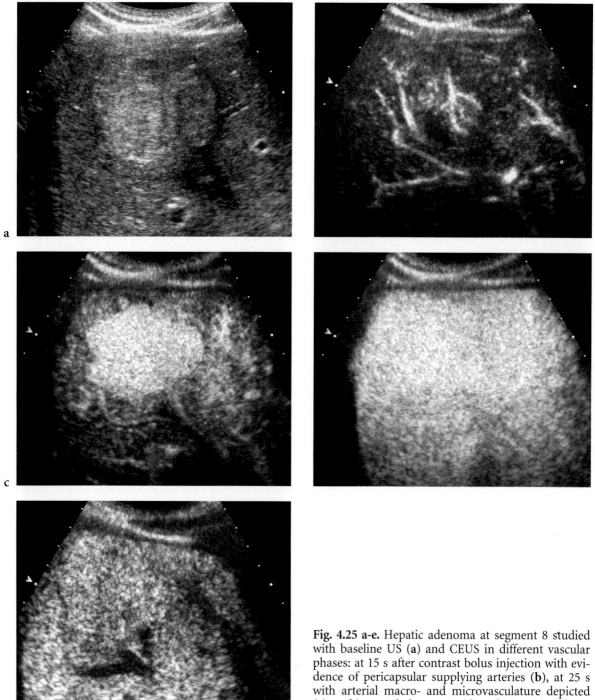

Fig. 4.25 a-e. Hepatic adenoma at segment 8 studied with baseline US (**a**) and CEUS in different vascular phases: at 15 s after contrast bolus injection with evidence of pericapsular supplying arteries (**b**), at 25 s with arterial macro- and microvasculature depicted (**c**), and in portal phase at 60 (**d**) and 180 s (**e**) with enhancement level equal to that of the surrounding normal liver parenchyma

Contrast-enhanced harmonic US (CEUS) allows depiction of the characteristic vascular behavior of hepatic adenomas. Early and homogeneous enhancement of nonhemorrhagic, nonnecrotic portions of the tumor is seen during the arterial phase (Fig. 4.24b). Identification of peritumoral feeding vessels is easier than with color Doppler and is crucial for the CEUS diagnosis of this disease. Pericapsular feeding blood vessels are best visualized in early arterial phase, particularly if a higher mechanical index (0.4–0.5) is employed (Fig. 4.24c). In late arterial and early portal phases, the contrast washout of HAs is initially faster than the progressive wash-in of the surrounding liver parenchyma. Consequently, the tumor remains slightly hypoechoic compared to the adjacent non-neoplastic liver (Fig. 4.24d). In late portal and sinusoidal phases, the tumor has usually the same vascular behavior of the surrounding liver parenchyma, being barely perceptible against the background of the enhanced liver tissue (Fig. 4.25).

These features of HA on CEUS strictly resemble those of contrast-enhanced helical computed tomography (CT) and magnetic resonance imaging (MRI). At contrast-enhanced CT, adenomas enhance early and homogeneously becoming moderately hyperattenuating in relation to the surrounding liver in the arterial phase. Peripheral enhancement corresponds to subcapsular feeding vessels. Adenomas then rapidly dismiss contrast becoming nearly isodense to the enhanced liver parenchyma (and therefore barely conspicuous) in the portal and delayed phases (Fig. 4.24e,f). In large tumors heterogeneity of the enhancement is due to areas of fat deposition, hemorrhage and necrosis (*Ichikawa 2000*). The same enhancement pattern observed with multiphasic helical CT applies to dynamic gadolinium-enhanced MRI (Fig. 4.24g), its most typical features being the early arterial enhancement due to hypervascularity (Fig. 4.24h), and rapid washout. Uptake of hepatobiliary MR contrast agents is due to hepatocellular nature of liver adenomas and may help in correct characterization (*Bartolozzi 2001*). Sometimes a low-signal peripheral rim is detectable and corresponds to the fibrous capsule (*Chung 1995*).

References

Bartolozzi C, Cioni D, Donati F, Lencioni R (2001) Focal liver lesions: MR imaging-pathologic correlation. Eur Radiol 11:1374-1388

Chung KY, Mayo-Smith WW, Saini S, et al (1995) Hepatocellular adenoma: MR imaging features with pathologic correlation. AJR 165:303-308

Golli M, Van Nhieu JT, Mathieu D, et al (1994) Hepatocellular adenoma: color Doppler US and pathologic correlations. Radiology 190:741-744

Grazioli L, Federle MP, Ichikawa T, et al (2000) Liver adenomatosis: clinical, histopathologic and imaging findings in 15 patients. Radiology 216:395-402

Ichikawa T, Federle MP, Grazioli L, Nalesnik M (2000) Hepatocellular adenoma: multiphasic CT and histopathologic findings in 25 patients. Radiology 214:861-868

Ros PR, Menu Y, Vilgrain V, Mortele KJ, Terris B (2001) Liver neoplasms and tumor-like conditions. Eur Radiol 11 [Suppl 2] S145-S165

4.4
Macro- and Microcirculation of Focal Nodular Hyperplasia

E. LEEN

Focal nodular hyperplasia is a benign congenital harmatomatous lesion and is the second most common benign tumour of the liver; it also represents about 4% of all primary hepatic tumors in the paediatric population.

They consist of abnormally arranged hepatocytes, Kupffer cells, bile duct elements and vascularised fibrous septae. They appear as multiple nodules separated by fibrous bands radiating from a central scar. The central or eccentric stellate scar contains fibrous tissue, bile ducts and thin-walled blood vessels; portal triads and central veins are, however, absent. The lesion is well circumscribed, non-encapsulated, with no calcification and is solitary in about 80% of cases.

Focal nodular hyperplasia occurs more commonly in young women than men with a 2-4-to-1 ratio and usually in their third to fifth decade. It has an increased incidence in those taking oral contraceptives. It is also associated with hepatic haemangiomas in about 23% of cases if oral contraceptives are used. Its detection is usually incidental as it is most often asymptomatic; vague abdominal pain is present in about 10% of patients due to the mass effect. More importantly it has no malignant potential; haemorrhage into the lesion is rare and management is therefore conservative.

On unenhanced conventional ultrasound, the lesion may be iso-, hypo- or hyperechoic; it may be difficult to delineate when it is iso-echoic but the diagnostic feature is the presence of the central scar, which may be found in 18% of cases. The central scar usually appears as a stellate or linear hypo- or anechoic area and the radiating fibrous septae may be more echogenic than the adjacent parenchymal tissue (Fig. 4.26). Focal nodular hyperplasia is a hypervascular lesion and unenhanced colour or power Doppler sonography may display the high-velocity Doppler signals within the central and radiating vessels.

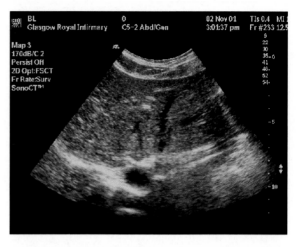

Fig. 4.26. Baseline ultrasound scan: Lesion is iso-echoic with a hypoechoic central scar

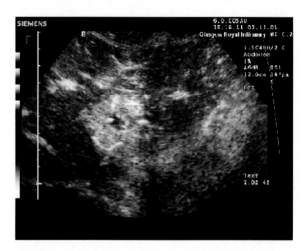

Fig. 4.27. Arterial phase of SonoVue administration: The focal nodular hyperplasia (FNH) enhances rapidly surrounded by the darker liver parenchyma, and the central artery adjacent to the lesion scar as well as the "spoke wheel" appearance is demonstrated

The hypervascularity of the lesion is easily demonstrated on SonoVue-enhanced ultrasound using any of the non-linear imaging modes at low mechanical index (MI) imaging. During the arterial phase, the lesional vessels are typically of the "stellate" or "spoke wheel" configuration, and, the lesion becomes homogenously hyper-echoic compared with the adjacent liver parenchyma within 15 s of the bolus injection of the contrast agent (Fig. 4.27). During the portal venous phase it remains hyperechoic against a background of enhanced

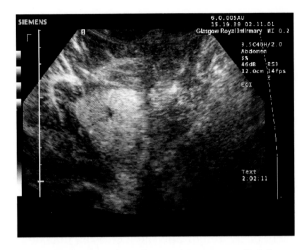

Fig. 4.28. Portal venous phase of SonoVue administration: There is further enhancement of the nodular lesion with the hypoechoic central scar standing out

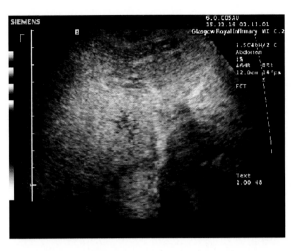

Fig. 4.29. Sinusoidal phase: There is as much contrast uptake within the lesion as in the surrounding liver parenchyma and the delineation of the lesion becomes less clear. The hypoechoic central scar is still clearly visible

normal liver tissue (Fig. 4.28) and gradually the lesion becomes isoechoic to the adjacent liver through to the later phase. Contrast is still held up homogenously within the lesion in the late sinusoidal phase (Fig. 4.29). During both the arterial and portal phases of the contrast injection, the central scar stands out easily as a hypo- or anechoic area within the hyperechoic lesion (*Leen 2001*). As with agents with tissue-specific affinity, there is uptake of the contrast in the late phase and again the central scar is easily depicted within the hyperechoic tumour (*Dill-Macky et al, 2002*). Given the clinical history, a definitive diagnosis can be made in the majority (if not all) of the patients.

References

Dill-Macky MJ, Burns PN, Khalili K, Wilson SR (2002) Focal hepatic masses: enhancement patterns with SHU 508A and pulse-inversion US. Radiology 222:95-102

Leen E (2001) The role of contrast enhanced ultrasound in the characterisation of focal liver lesions. Eur Radiol 11 [Suppl 3]:E27-34

4.5
Other Benign Lesions and Pseudolesions

L. Solbiati, V. Kirn, L. Cova

4.5.1
Inflammatory Pseudotumor of the Liver

Inflammatory pseudotumor of the liver (IPTL) is an uncommon, benign hepatic disease characterized by a well-circumscribed mass consisting of chronic inflammatory cell infiltration and fibrosis (*Nam 1996; Coffin 1991*). IPTL is more frequent in the male sex. Patients usually present with systemic complaint consisting of fever, malaise and weight loss, together with upper abdominal pain (*Horiuchi 1990; Zamir 1998*). Laboratory data are usually consistent with systemic inflammation, while serum alpha-fetoprotein levels are normal.

The etiology of this disease is still controversial: some authors suggest that micro-organisms from food, cholangitis or chronic intra-abdominal infection ascending by the portal blood stream may seed in the hepatic parenchyma, eliciting an inflammatory lesion with obliterating phlebitis (*Horiuchi 1990*).

IPTL is usually (but not always) solitary and may frequently reach fairly large size (over 5 cm).

Sonography usually shows large, inhomogeneous hypoechoic masses, with multiple thin septae and increased through-transmission (*Nam 1996; Liessi 1995*), but this "mosaic-like" sonographic appearance is not specific.

On contrast-enhanced computed tomography (CT) in portal phase IPTL shows a variable degree of hyperdensity in respect to surrounding hepatic parenchyma and evident heterogeneity, with presence of multiple enhancing areas intermingled with unenhanced ones (*Fukuya 1994; Kelekis 1995*). Peripheral enhancement on delayed-phase CT may also be found, probably because of extravascular contrast accumulation in fibrotic components of the mass with delayed washout (*Fukuya 1994*) (Fig. 4.30f). It is likely that higher echogenicity and higher attenuation areas correspond to fibrosis sites, while lower echogenicity and attenuation areas correspond to sites of predominantly cellular infiltration.

Contrast-enhanced ultrasound (CEUS) shows, in arterial phase, only peripheral feeding arteries with a rim-like appearance (Fig. 4.30b). In early portal phase, progressive enhancement of the solid portion of the mass occurs with centrifugal development. At this time (30–40 s after contrast bolus administration), most of the tumor (apart from the central fluid collection) shows an enhancement level equivalent to that of the surrounding liver parenchyma, while the thick, rim-like outer portion representing perilesional fibrotic tissue remains unenhanced (Fig. 4.30c). Subsequently, at 45–70 s, the decreasing enhancement of the tumor and the increasing uptake of the perilesional fibrosis parallel and the two portions become indistinguishable (Fig. 4.30d).

4.5.2
Hepatic Tuberculoma

Hepatosplenic tuberculosis is common in miliary tuberculosis and is found in 70%-80% of autopsy cases with disseminated pulmonary tuberculosis (*Thoeni 1979*). Infection probably spreads to the liver from para-aortic to portal nodes via the portal vein or hepatic artery. Hepatic tubercolomas may be multiple or single and are usually small. Liver size and texture may greatly vary from case to case (*Hulnick 1985; Brauner 1989*).

On baseline US, either single or (more commonly) multiple hypoechoic, well-marginated lesions are generally seen, scattered throughout the liver (*Brauner 1989; Levine 1990*). In some cases, tuberculomas have ill-defined margins and are not clearly identifiable against the background of liver parenchyma with inhomogeneous echotexture (Fig. 4.31a). Occasionally, tuberculomas may appear hyperechoic, with or without calcifications.

On CT, tuberculomas present as solid, hypodense, well-marginated and heterogeneous masses with low attenuation values ranging from 14 to 45 HU (*Brauner 1989; Levine 1990*). After contrast administration, the rim of the lesion enhances moderately while the low-density center remains unchanged .

Magnetic resonance imaging (MRI) of the liver demonstrates hypodense nodules with a hypointense rim on T1-weighted images, and isointense and hyperintense nodules with a

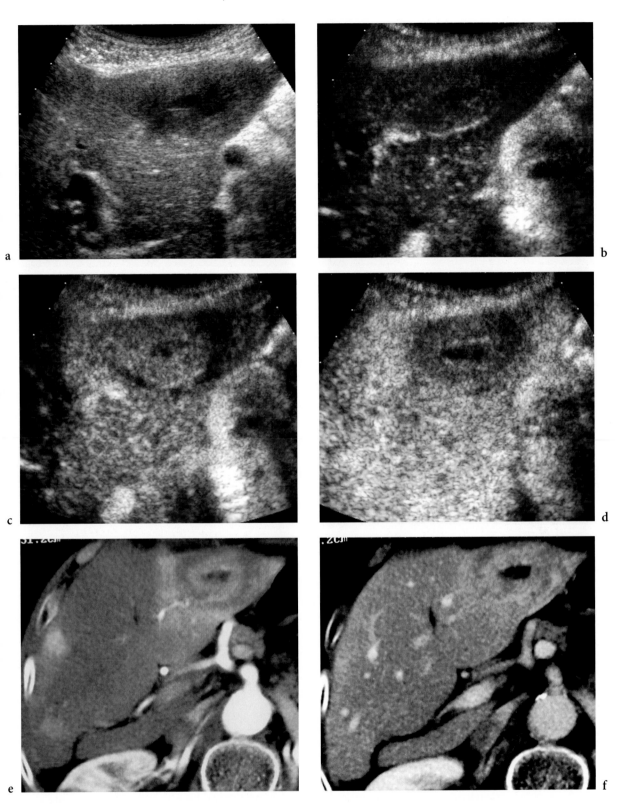

Fig. 4.30 a-f. Inflammatory pseudotumor at segment 3. The 5-cm mass (**a**) has a central fluid collection and a solid peripheral portion. The enhancement pattern in arterial phase at 20 s (**b**), early portal phase at 35 s (**c**) and full portal phase at 60 s (**d**) shows a progressive centrifugal increase and it is very similar to that of contrast-enhanced helical CT in arterial (**e**) and portal venous (**f**) phases

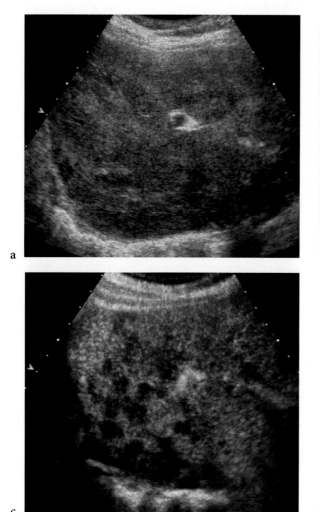

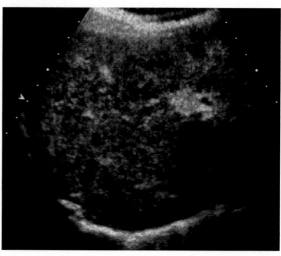

Fig. 4.31 a-c. Hepatic tuberculosis. On baseline sonography (**a**), liver echotexture is markedly inhomogeneous and tubercolomas are not easily identifiable. On CEUS, no focal enhancing lesions are depicted in arterial phase (**b**), whereas hypoechoic, poorly enhancing and irregularly shaped tubercolomas are clearly identifiable in full portal venous phase, at 90 s after contrast bolus injection (**c**)

less intense rim on T2-weighted images.

With contrast-enhanced US, tuberculomas do not show any selective enhancement in arterial phase (Fig. 4.31b), while they are clearly detectable in full and delayed portal phases as poorly enhancing, hypoechoic, well-marginated nodules with irregular shape and often confluent to form larger focal lesions (Fig. 4.31c).

These imaging features are not specific to hepatic tuberculosis and therefore, if clinical findings are not highly significant, final diagnosis has to be established by means of percutaneous biopsy (*Akhan 2002*).

4.5.3
Focal Fatty Changes

Liver steatosis can result from decreased hepatic clearance of fatty acids from hepatocellular injury or from increased production or mobilization of fatty acids. Common etiologies include alcohol, diabetes, obesity and drugs. Fatty changes may be either homogeneously diffused throughout the liver, or "geographically" distributed or, more rarely, may present as single well-demarcated foci. Histologic examination of the focal fatty lesions shows an amount of lipidic vacuoles present only inside the areas (Fig. 4.32h) and absent in the adjacent liver parenchyma (Fig. 4.32g).

Focal fatty deposits are frequently encountered in sonographic studies of the liver. They usually appear as hyperechoic liver segments ("segmental" distribution) or zones ("geographic" pattern) or oval to rounded nodules, up to 3 cm in size. This "pseudonodular" pattern is sometimes very questionable, particularly in patients with history of neoplastic disease and not previously having undergone imaging studies of the liver.

On CT, fatty "pseudonodules" may be questionable, too, being difficult to distinguish from primary or metastatic liver neoplasms in some occurrences (*Kroncke 2000*). On unenhanced CT, they appear as areas of low attenuation, with no selective enhancement in arterial phase after contrast administration (Fig. 4.32e) and hypodense pattern in portal venous phase (Fig. 4.32f). Both on US and CT, focal fatty changes do not show any mass effect on the adjacent parenchyma, and vascular structures can be seen coursing in a normal pattern through the fatty areas (*Apecella 2000*). However, note should be made of the very rare cases of metastatic lesions transversed by vascular structures (*Anthony 1978*).

The hyperintense pattern on T1-weighted MRI (*Kawamori 1996*) may be the clue for diagnosis in doubtful cases, but, before moving to MRI, CEUS can be performed with second-generation contrast agents and harmonic imaging. With CEUS it can easily be shown that even very questionable nodular fatty changes on B-mode US (Fig. 4.32a,b) have typically no arterial enhancement (Fig. 4.32c), whereas in portal venous phase they enhance with speed and intensity exactly equal to the surrounding normal liver, becoming absolutely indistinguishable (Fig. 4.32d). Consequently, CEUS may be suggested as the first imaging modality after baseline US, before moving to CT, MRI or even aspiration biopsy.

4.5.4
Skip Areas in Diffuse Steatosis

Focal spared areas, also known as "skip areas", are frequently encountered in diffuse fatty liver. They are typically located along the hepatic hilum or around the gallbladder in most cases. This peculiar distribution is due to the fact that in these areas, "nonportal" splanchnic venous supply replaces the absent or reduced portal venous blood flow. As a consequence, these zones undergo less intrahepatocytic deposition of triglycerides than the surrounding liver tissue (*Rubaltelli 2002*). Another characteristic location of focal sparing is around liver tumors, due to the local deficit of portal venous flow (*Itai 2002*).

Histologic examination of focal spared areas shows normal liver parenchyma.

On baseline sonography, skip areas usually appear as hypoechoic foci with ill-defined margins, in bright fatty livers, typically located in the above-mentioned liver zones (*Rubaltelli 2002*) (Fig. 4.33a). When this is the sonographic pattern, no further diagnostic assessment is needed.

In rare occurrences, however, skip areas may present as rounded, "nodular" foci, up to 2–2.5 cm in size, either single or multiple and located in different liver segments (*Rubaltelli 2002*) (Fig. 4.34a). Particularly if this pattern occurs in patients with questionable clinical findings or history of neoplastic disease, further diagnostic work-up (CT, MRI and/or aspiration biopsy) is absolutely required. Currently, CEUS can be usefully employed as first-line imaging modality in these cases, being able to provide quick, reliable and inexpensive diagnoses. On CEUS, in fact, skip areas with both typical and atypical "pseudonodular" sonographic pattern show the same unequivocal enhancement findings: lack of hyperechoic foci in arterial phase (Figs. 4.33b, 4.34b) and homogeneous enhancement, of the same intensity of liver parenchyma, in portal venous phase (Figs. 4.33c, 4.34c) with complete "disappearance" of skip areas. An equal enhancement pattern is shown by contrast-enhanced CT (*Paulson 1993*) (Fig. 4.34d,e).

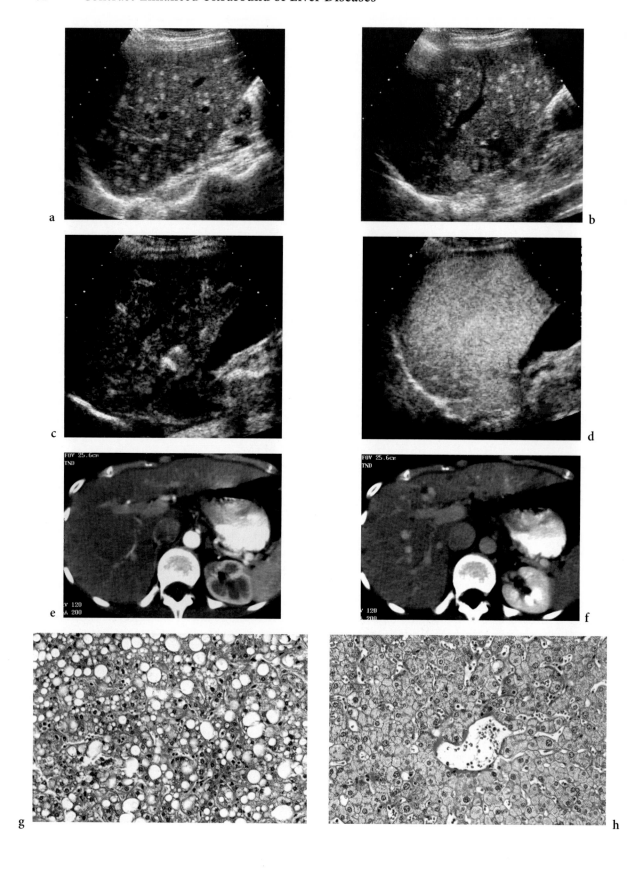

◄ **Fig. 4.32 a-h.** In this 38-year-old female patient complaining of aspecific pain in her right upper quadrant and never previously having undergone any imaging study of the liver, baseline US discovers multiple hyperechoic, rounded and well-demarcated nodules scattered throughout the liver (**a**, **b**). CEUS shows no enhancing areas in arterial phase (**c**) and homogeneous enhancement in portal venous phase (**d**) with complete disappearance of any focal change, thus favoring the diagnosis of fatty "pseudonodular" changes. Contrast-enhanced CT confirms the lack of hyperenhancing nodules in arterial phase (**e**), but shows many hypodense nodules in portal phase (**f**), raising the suspicion of metastatic deposits. Sonographically guided aspiration biopsy is subsequently performed both into the hyperechoic foci (obtaining fatty liver tissue) (**g**) and in the normal liver parenchyma where normal hepatocytes are found (**h**)

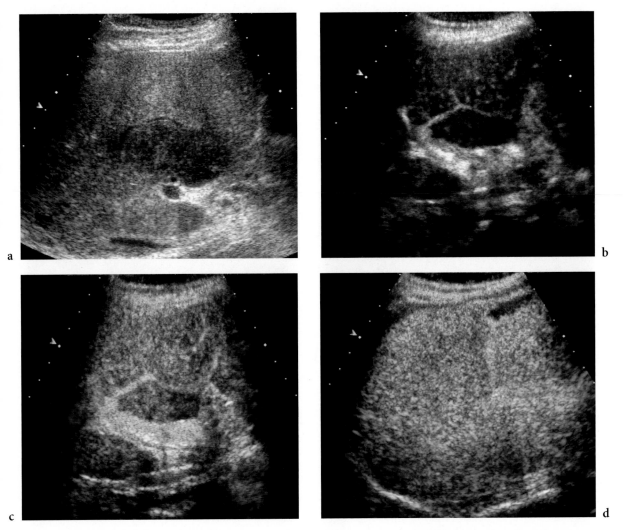

Fig. 4.33 a-d. Typical skip area at segment 4 in fatty liver. Hypoechoic pattern on baseline US (**a**). On CEUS, no enhancement in arterial phase (**b**) and progressive enhancement in early (**c**) and delayed (**d**) portal phase, with intensity comparable to that of liver parenchyma

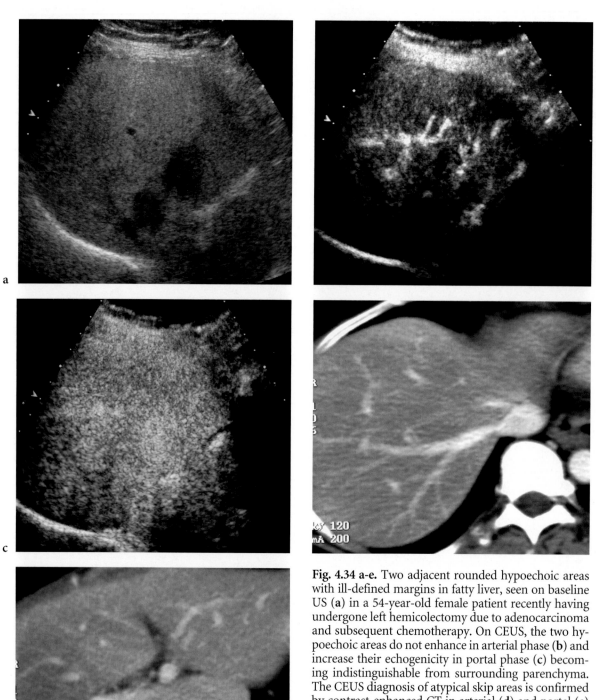

Fig. 4.34 a-e. Two adjacent rounded hypoechoic areas with ill-defined margins in fatty liver, seen on baseline US (**a**) in a 54-year-old female patient recently having undergone left hemicolectomy due to adenocarcinoma and subsequent chemotherapy. On CEUS, the two hypoechoic areas do not enhance in arterial phase (**b**) and increase their echogenicity in portal phase (**c**) becoming indistinguishable from surrounding parenchyma. The CEUS diagnosis of atypical skip areas is confirmed by contrast-enhanced CT in arterial (**d**) and portal (**e**) phases : the two foci are isodense with the surrounding parenchyma in both vascular phases

References

Akhan O, Pringot J (2002) Imaging of abdominal tuberculosis. Eur Radiol 12:321-323

Anthony P, Ishak K, Nayak N (1978) The morphology of cirrhosis. Recommendation on definition, nomenclature and classification by a working group sponsored by WHO. J Clin Pathol 31:395-401

Apecella PL, Mirowitz SA, Weinreb JC (1994) Extension of vessel through hepatic neoplasms: MR and CT findings. Radiology 191:135-140

Brauner M, Buffard MD, Jaentils V, Legrand I (1989) Sonography and computed tomography of macroscopic tuberculosis of the liver. J Clin Ultrasound 17:563-568

Coffin CM, Watterson J, Priest JR, Dehner LP (1995) Extrapulmonary inflammatory myofibroblastic tumor (inflammatory pseudotumor). A clinicopathologic and immunohistochemical study of 84 cases. Am J Surg Pathol 19:859-872

Fukuya T, Honda H, Matsumata T, et al (1994) Diagnosis of inflammatory pseudotumor of the liver: value of CT. AJR 163:1087-1091

Horiuchi R, Uchida T, Kojima T (1990) Inflammatory pseudotumor of the liver. Clinicopathologic study and review of the literature. Cancer 65:1583-1590

Hulnick DH, Megibow AJ, Naidich DP, Hilton S, Cho KC, Balthazar EJ (1985) Abdominal tuberculosis : CT evaluation. Radiology 157:199-204

Itai Y, Saida Y (2002) Pitfalls in liver imaging. Eur Radiol 12:1162-1174

Kawamori Y, Matsui O, Takahashi S, Kadoya M, Takashima T, Miyayama S (1996) Focal hepatic fatty infiltration in the posterior edge of the medial segment associated with aberrant gastric venous drainage: CT, US, and MR findings. J Comput Assist Tomogr 20:356-359

Kelekis NL, Warshauer DM, Semelka RC, Eisenberg LB, Woosley JT (1995) Inflammatory pseudotumor of the liver: appearance on contrast enhanced helical CT and dynamic MR images. J Magn Reson Imaging 5:551-553

Kroncke TJ, Taupitz M, Kivelitz D (2000) Multifocal nodular fatty infiltration of the liver mimicking metastatic disease on CT: imaging findings using MR imaging. Eur Radiol 10:1095-1100

Levine C (1990) Primary macronodular hepatic tuberculosis: US and CT appearances. Gastrointest Radiol 15:307-309

Liessi G, Mastropasqua G, Spaliviero B, Butini R, Pavanello M (1995) Pseudotumore del fegato: imaging con ecografia, Tomografia Computerizzata e Risonanza Magnetica in un caso. Radiol Med 89:545-548

Nam KJ, Kang HK, Lim JH (1996) Inflammatory pseudotumor of the liver: CT and sonographic features. AJR 167:485-487

Paulson EK, Baker ME, Spritzer CE, Leder RA, Gulliver DJ, Meyers WC (1993) Focal fatty infiltration: a cause of nontumourous defects in the left hepatic lobe during CT arterial portography. J Comput Assist Tomogr 17:590-595

Rubaltelli L, Savastano S, Khadivi J, Stramare R, Tregnaghi A, Da Pian P (2002) Targetlike appearance of pseudotumors in segment IV of the liver on sonography. AJR 178(1):75-77

Thoeni RF, Margulis AR (1979) Gastrointestinal tuberculosis: Semin Roentgenol 14:283-294

Zamir D, Jarchwksy J, Singer C, et al (1998) Inflammatory pseudotumor of the liver. A rare entity and a diagnostic challenge. Am J Gastroenterol 38:1538-1540

4.6
Hepatocellular Carcinoma and Dysplastic Lesions

L. SOLBIATI, M. TONOLINI, L. COVA

4.6.1
Introduction and Epidemiology

Hepatocellular carcinoma (HCC) is the most common primary liver malignancy. Its incidence is currently increasing worldwide and reaches an estimated 1,000,000 new cases per year. Striking geographical differences are observed for its occurrence: the highest incidence rates of this tumor are found in South-East Asia, China and sub-Saharan Africa. Areas of low incidence (<5 new cases/100,000 inhabitants/year) include northern Europe and America, whereas Mediterranean countries are in an intermediate position (10-20 cases/100,000/year). This peculiar distribution is related to the etiology of the disease: in countries with low to intermediate incidence, most cases can be attributed to chronic hepatitis B and C virus infections. Conversely, environmental and dietary factors such as aflatoxins play a major role in Africa and Asia. HCC most often occurs in association with cirrhosis or chronic hepatitis. All individuals with chronic liver disease are considered at increased risk of HCC occurrence. World-prevalent hepatitis B and C virus infections and alcoholism currently account for the majority of HCC cases; in particular, hepatitis C virus (HCV) is becoming the leading cause. Among less common causes are hemochromatosis and Wilson disease.

Given the wide range of treatment options currently available for cirrhotic patients affected with HCC, including surgical resection, transplantation, transarterial chemoembolization (TACE) and percutaneous methods such as ethanol injection, laser and radiofrequency (RF) ablation, timely detection and accurate staging are mandatory so as to determine the best therapeutic outcome.

In cirrhotic patients, the development of HCC may be heralded by abrupt worsening of the clinical picture and liver function tests. Advanced HCC manifests itself with upper abdominal pain, weight loss, ascites and possibly jaundice. Signs and symptoms of a small tumor are usually indistinguishable from those of underlying cirrhosis. Currently, in most developed countries, HCC is usually detected at an early stage by close surveillance of high-risk patients. Follow-up with liver ultrasound and serum alpha-fetoprotein levels every 4-6 months enables earlier detection and prompt treatment of this cancer.

The clinical course shows significant variability, and prognosis is affected by tumor features (including number and size of nodules, presence of a capsule, degree of differentiation, vascular invasion) as well as severity of the underlying chronic liver disease and portal hypertension.

4.6.2
Pathology and Hepatocarcinogenesis

Liver cirrhosis is defined by disruption of hepatic architecture with diffuse development of hepatocellular regenerative nodules (RNs) surrounded by fibrous septa. Cirrhosis may be classified according to the size of the dominant regenerative nodule pattern as micro- (<3 mm), macronodular (>3 mm) or mixed. Large RNs at least 5mm in diameter are called macroregenerative nodules. RNs rarely exceed 20 mm: when larger nodules are present in cirrhosis, they are invariably dysplastic.

Pathology studies have identified a spectrum of nodular hepatocellular lesions that occupy an intermediate position between regenerative nodules and well-differentiated HCC. Dysplastic nodules (DNs) are lesions arising in the cirrhotic liver and may be single or multiple. Their histological features are cellular atypia without frank malignant changes and development of small arteries without accompanying bile ducts (unpaired or non-triadal). The premalignant nature of DNs has been extensively demonstrated. Dysplastic nodules are pathologically identified at about 8-10 mm and may sometimes reach 15-20 mm.

"Small" HCCs (the cut-off set at 30 mm has been lowered to 20 mm) are generally well-differentiated. As they reach this size range, their growth pattern becomes distinctly nodular, making their detection easier. At histology, portal tracts disappear and the number of unpaired arteries further increases.

It is currently accepted that hepatic carcinogenesis in the cirrhotic liver is a stepwise process (*Efremidis and Hytiroglou 2002*). The multistep model involves the transition from frankly benign nodules (macro-RNs) to premalignant low-grade and high-grade dysplasia, to early well-differentiated HCC and finally to overt HCC. During this process, intranodular hemodynamic changes also occur : whereas regenerative and dysplastic lesions maintain portal blood supply, development of HCC means the appearance of arterial neovascularization (*Kudo 1999*). The hypervascularity of HCC in cirrhosis is due to neoangiogenesis occurring in a background of arterialization of the liver parenchyma and capillarization of the sinusoids. The progressive obstruction to portal flow due to the disruption of normal liver architecture and replacement with fibrosis causes the liver to become progressively more dependent on arterial blood supply. At the same time the sinusoids undergo "capillarization" developing basement membranes and lose endothelial "fenestrae." In the meantime, neoangiogenesis takes place in the form of unpaired (non-triadal) arteries during the evolution of nodules to HCC through a balance of angiogenic factors elaborated by tumoral cells.

As the tumor grows from a small HCC, progressive de-differentiation occurs. Lower histologic grade cancerous tissue proliferates within the nodule (so-called nodule-in-nodule appearance), gradually replaces the well-differentiated HCC and starts to grow expansively (*Efremidis and Hytigolou 2002; Kojiro and Nakashima 1999*). The arterial supply of HCC increases in parallel to a size and grading of the tumor, whereas the portal supply decreases during the earlier steps of carcinogenesis.

HCC frequently occurs multicentrically, either synchronous or metachronous (*Kojiro and Nakashima 1999*). On gross pathology, overt HCC may be classified as expansive (nodular or multifocal), massive infiltrating or diffuse. Macroscopically, the tumor nodules may be homogeneous or may have necrotic and hemorrhagic changes. Unusual histologic features include fatty metamorphosis, necro-

sis, abundant fibrosclerotic stroma and even more rarely calcifications and copper deposition.

Pathology demonstrates a fibrous capsule in 50%-60% of cases. Small, well-differentiated HCCs (<3 cm) are unencapsulated, whereas expansive-type medium-sized HCCs usually possess a well-defined capsule.

Portal invasion occurs in a significant proportion of patients (up to 65% in autopsy series). Venous extension is more frequent in large, infiltrating and/or poorly differentiated hepatocellular carcinomas. According to pathologists, multicentric forms of HCC may be explained by portal dissemination.

4.6.3
Unenhanced Sonography

Ultrasound (US) is by far the most common examination in screening of patients at high risk of developing hepatocellular carcinomas such as alcoholic, hepatitis B and C, and hemochromatosis patients, thanks to its low cost, nearly universal availability and repeatability. Among its drawbacks are dependancy on operator expertise and inherent limitations due to patient body habitus, bowel gas distention and inhomogeneity of liver parenchyma.

The US appearance of HCC is usually nonspecific and varies depending on the size of the tumor, the fat content, degree of differentiation, presence of scarring or necrosis. Commonly, small tumors (<3 cm in diameter) are hypoechoic and uniform in appearance, but some lesions may appear hyperechoic due to fatty change. They may show irregular margins or have a well-defined hypoechoic rim corresponding to the presence of a pseudocapsule. US has limited value in demonstration of fibrous capsules. Larger HCCs are usually heterogeneous with mixed hyper- and hypoechogenicity.

Doppler studies may be useful in characterization of HCC. Characteristic hypervascularity of HCC manifests itself with intratumoral pulsatile flow on color/power Doppler with high-velocity systolic intralesional signals. The "basket" pattern of vessels surrounding and penetrating or a "vessel-within-the-tumor" pattern are often visible on color Doppler in

HCCs but in RNs and DNs. However, they have not been proved to affect sensitivity for the detection of HCCs.

Given a wide range of technology (conventional sonography and Doppler), the reported detection rate of HCCs measuring less than 2 cm in diameter has been variable, ranging from 46% to 95% (*Choi et al. 1989; Matsui and Itai 1992*), with accurate detection of 82%–93% of HCCs measuring between 2 and 3 cm. For HCCs smaller than 1 cm, the detection rate by US is considerably lower and ranges between 13% and 37% (*Matsui and Itai 1992*).

Furthermore, the US appearance of a small HCC (Fig. 4.35c) is usually indistinguishable on conventional US from a regenerative or dysplastic nodule (Fig. 4.35a) : the detection of a small nodule in a cirrhotic patient may represent a hyperplastic, dysplastic or tumoral nodule. Thus, the identification of focal abnormalities usually leads to further investigations, like computed tomography (CT), magnetic resonance imaging (MRI) and sometimes biopsy.

US has limited value in staging of HCC. Multifocal tumors and daughter (satellite) nodules are two common features of HCCs, but nonintraoperative US usually underestimates the number of both multicentric and daughter HCCs. US and color Doppler may usually detect tumor extension into the portal trunk and main branches or hepatic veins, although detection of segmental or subsegmental portal thrombosis is limited. Confident characterization of malignancy is possible only when color Doppler detects pulsatile arterial flow signals within the thrombus.

4.6.4
Contrast-Enhanced Ultrasound

Since the most important feature that allows characterization of a nodule in cirrhosis and detection of HCC is its peculiar blood supply, contrast-enhanced ultrasound (CEUS) may play an important role in this disease. After initial experiences using high-mechanical index (MI) intermittent ultrasonic scans with first generation contrast agents (*Bertolotto et al. 2000; Blomley et al. 2001; Choi et al. 2002; Dill-Macky et al. 2002*), continuous-mode low-MI

harmonic US with second-generation contrast agents (like SonoVue™, Bracco, Milan, Italy) is currently the sonographic modality with the highest sensitivity for detection, characterization and staging of HCC. Thanks to the possibility of studying adequately the arterial phase (15–25 s following the injection), the portal phase (45–90 s) and the "sinusoidal phase" (90-240 s), HCCs can be detected and characterized with high accuracy using CEUS (*Numata 2001, Solbiati 2000; Wilson 2000*).

First of all, CEUS is extremely helpful for differentiating macroregenerative and dysplastic nodules from HCCs. Macroregenerative nodules are rarely seen on baseline US when they reach a sufficient size (8-10 mm) and distort liver margins.

On CEUS they do not show any selective enhancement in arterial phase, while in portal and sinusoidal phases macro-RNs enhance homogeneously and to the same degree as the surrounding fibrotic parenchyma, from which they cannot be differentiated.

A similar enhancement pattern is always shown by dysplastic nodules which often appear as slightly hypoechoic focal lesions on baseline US, not clearly differentiable from early HCCs. Therefore, the first goal of CEUS in cirrhotic patients is the differentiation of HCCs from RNs and DNs (Fig. 4.35).

On CEUS, the characteristic pattern of HCC is represented by an intense and fast peak of enhancement in the arterial phase (from approximately 20 s after contrast injection), followed by a relatively quick "wash out", starting at the beginning of the portal phase and quickly increasing towards the sinusoidal phase, when the tumor appears markedly hypoechoic compared to the surrounding liver parenchyma (*Leen et al. 2001; Solbiati et al. 2000; Solbiati et al. 2001; Tanaka et al. 2001; Wilson et al. 2000*) (Fig. 4.36) .

Chaotic peritumoral and intralesional tortuous "corkscrew"/"s"-shaped vessels may be seen in the arterial phase (Fig. 4.37) as well as during the overlap with the portal phase. Vascular lakes subsequently appear as dense focal areas of increased echogenicity (Fig. 4.38). Feeding vessels, which are not appreciated on conventional colorDoppler US or contrast-enhanced CT, are identified in most cases. Unlike

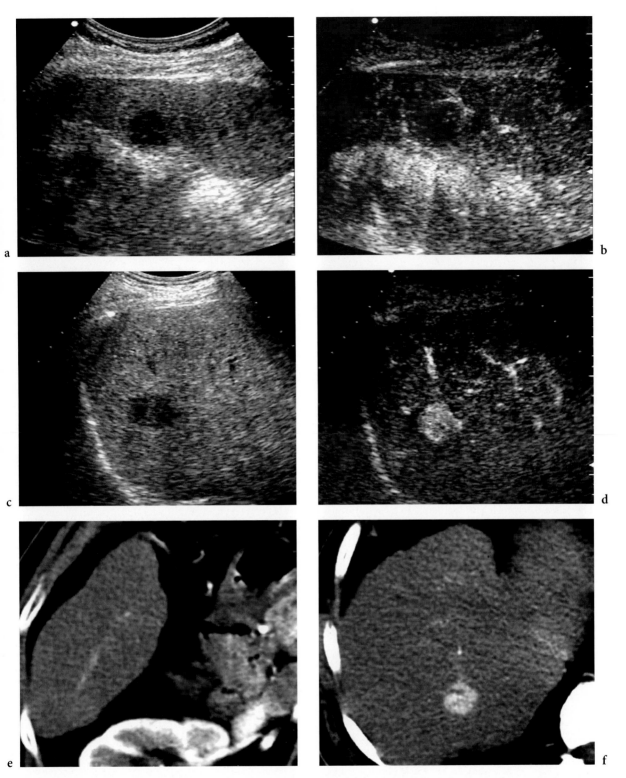

Fig. 4.35 a-f. Cirrhotic patient with two hypoechoic nodules detected on baseline US. The 15-mm lesion at segment 6 (**a**) does not show any enhancement in arterial phase (**b**) and remains isoechoic in portal phase, while the 25-mm nodule at segment 8 (**c**) has marked arterial enhancement, becoming hyperechoic (**d**) and subsequently has a fast washout, becoming hypoechoic in portal phase. On contrast-enhanced helical CT, the first lesion (dysplastic nodule) is undetectable in arterial phase, due to lack of enhancement (**e**), while the nodule at segment 8 (HCC) is clearly hyperattenuating in the same phase (**f**)

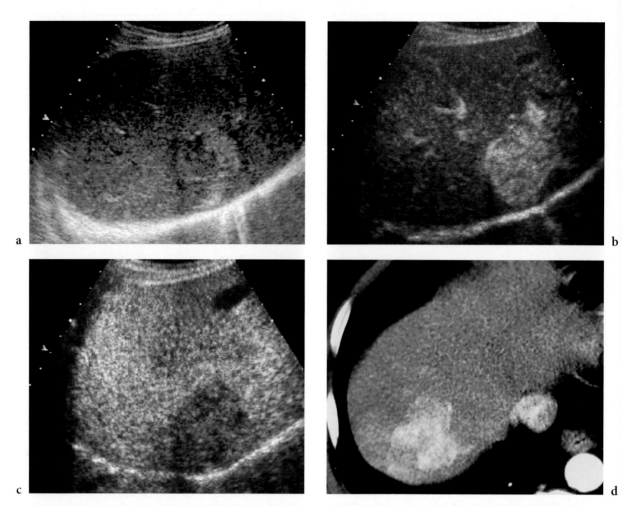

Fig. 4.36 a-d. 4-cm HCC at segment 7 in a cirrhotic patient. The lesion is typically slightly hyperechoic on baseline US (**a**), markedly hyperechoic during the arterial enhancement (**b**) and clearly hypoechoic in portal phase (90 s after contrast administration) (**c**). Contrast-enhanced helical CT in arterial phase (**d**) confirms the diagnosis of HCC

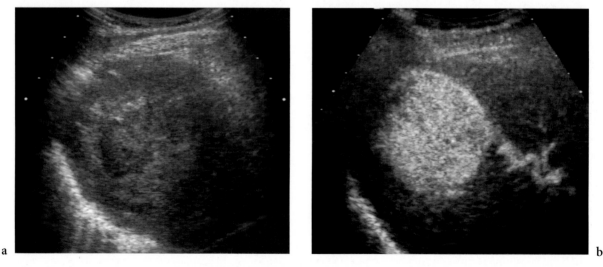

Fig. 4.37 a,b. Large HCC (6.5 cm) at segment 8 (**a**) with intense and homogeneous enhancement in arterial phase (**b**). The corkscrew-shaped large arterial blood vessel supplying the mass is clearly visible

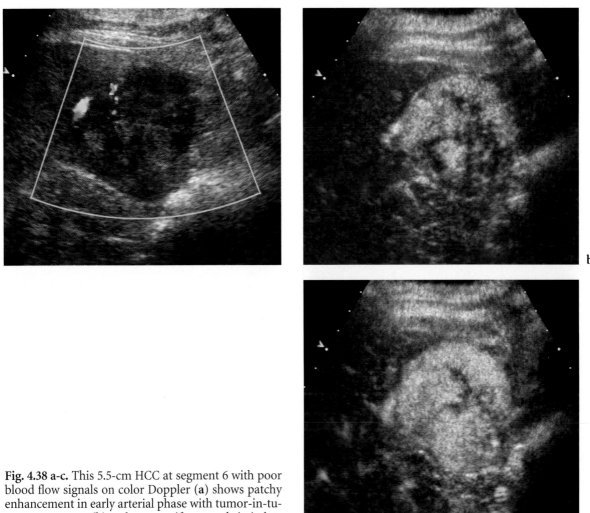

Fig. 4.38 a-c. This 5.5-cm HCC at segment 6 with poor blood flow signals on color Doppler (**a**) shows patchy enhancement in early arterial phase with tumor-in-tumor appearance (**b**) and more uniform wash-in in late arterial phase (**c**)

some benign liver tumors (like adenomas), pericapsular enhancement in arterial phase is never detected with CEUS, even in capsulated, expansive-type medium-sized HCCs .

This peculiar vascular pattern (well comparable to that achieved with contrast-enhanced CT and MR) (*Baron et al. 1996; Bartolozzi et al. 1999; Bluemke et al. 2000; Matsuo 2001*) is seen in 90%-96% of HCCs, almost independently of the histologic grade of malignancy. In particular, the fast arterial enhancement is routinely identifiable even in patients with slow hepatic circulation, thanks to the real-time visualization of the enhanced blood flow. In the early portal phase, most HCCs become undetectable due to the marked increase of liver enhancement and the reduction of liver-to-tumor en-

hancement ratio. In high-grade cirrhosis, the portal phase may be delayed and the liver parenchymal enhancement may appear less intense. Although SonoVue™ does not have any late liver parenchymal uptake, scans performed at 3–4 min after bolus administration ("sinusoidal phase") routinely show a persistent detectable sinusoidal enhancement of liver parenchyma, probably due to entrapment of microbubbles into the sinusoids, with HCCs manifesting as focal hypoechoic well-demarcated lesions (*Leen 2001*) (Fig. 4.39).

Consequently, in cirrhotic patients a hepatocellular nodule greater than 10 mm with different echogenicity on baseline US, which enhances on CEUS in the hepatic arterial phase and shows lack of enhancement in the portal

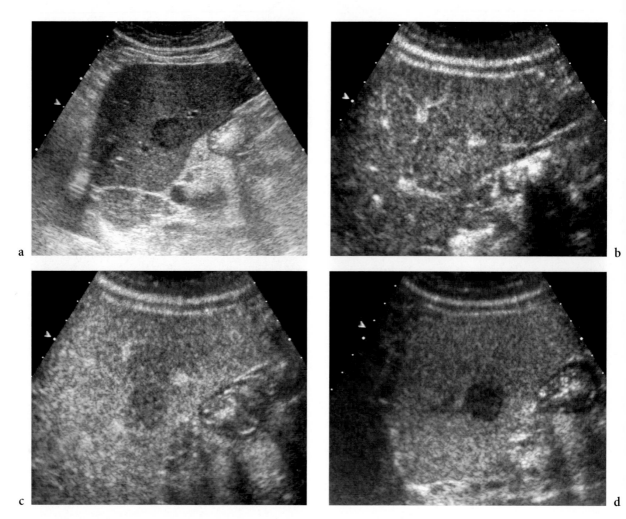

Fig. 4.39 a-d. In rare cases like this 1.8-cm HCC at segment 3 (**a**), on CEUS the arterial enhancement (**b**) is poor and the washout very fast, with hypoechoic pattern only 45 s after contrast administration (**c**). The mass is better identifiable as a markedly hypoechoic nodule in the sinusoidal phase (at 180 s) (**d**)

venous phase, has to be considered a small HCC. It is universally accepted that HCC can be diagnosed by means of biopsy or when a focal lesion of at least 2 cm in diameter shows evidence of hypervascularity on either imaging modality with or without raised (>400 ng/ml) serum alpha-fetoprotein levels (*Bruix* 2001). Therefore, CEUS with second-generation microbubbles can currently be included in the group of imaging modalities of crucial importance for the diagnosis of HCC.

In the remaining 4%–10% of HCCs, only heterogeneous weak enhancement (mostly with peripheral rim-like appearance) is identified on CEUS (Fig. 4.40). This occurs usually for largely necrotic HCCs and, less frequently,

for cancers with fatty changes. Since also contrast-enhanced CT and MRI show questionable inhomogeneous enhancement in most of these occurrences, biopsy is usually mandatory for the final diagnosis.

While the hypervascular pattern described above allows a reliable characterization of HCC in most cases, the major problem for CEUS remains the detection of HCC, particularly for lesions undetected on baseline US and/or for multifocal lesions (Fig. 4.41), given the need to explore thoroughly the entire liver parenchyma during the very short arterial phase duration. This may require more administrations of contrast agent (at least one for each lobe), good technical skill in performing

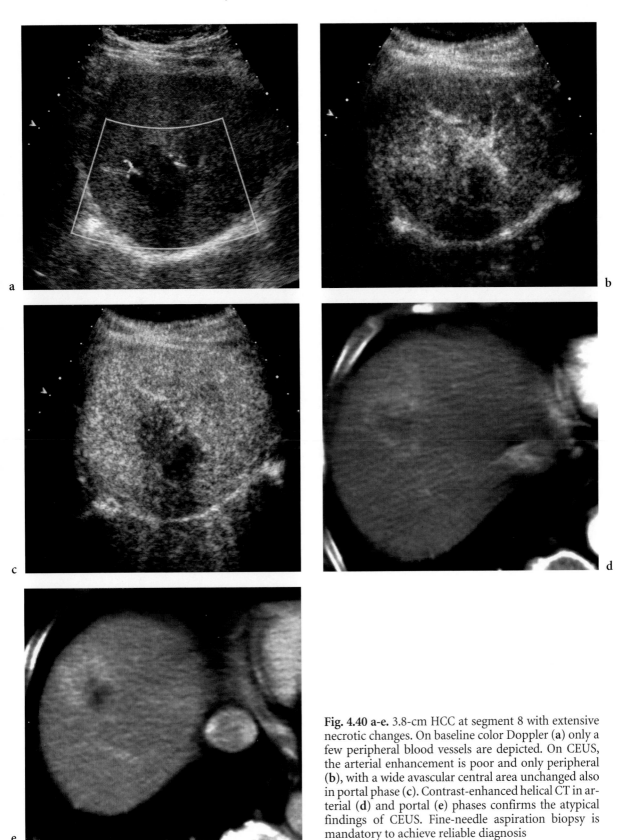

Fig. 4.40 a-e. 3.8-cm HCC at segment 8 with extensive necrotic changes. On baseline color Doppler (**a**) only a few peripheral blood vessels are depicted. On CEUS, the arterial enhancement is poor and only peripheral (**b**), with a wide avascular central area unchanged also in portal phase (**c**). Contrast-enhanced helical CT in arterial (**d**) and portal (**e**) phases confirms the atypical findings of CEUS. Fine-needle aspiration biopsy is mandatory to achieve reliable diagnosis

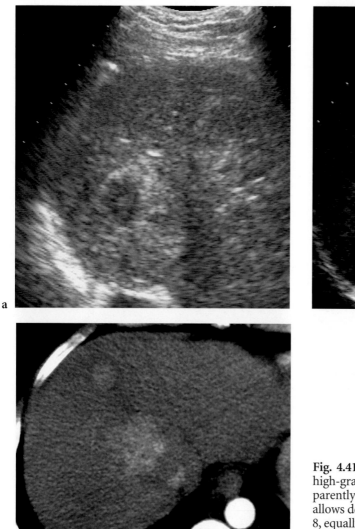

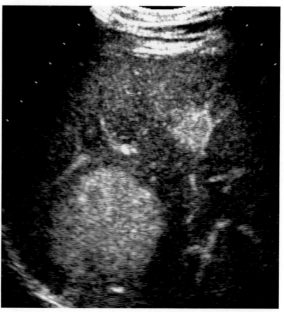

Fig. 4.41 a-c. a Multifocality detected with CEUS. In high-grade cirrhotic patient, baseline US depicts an apparently single HCC (5 cm) at segment 7, while CEUS allows detection of a second lesion (1.5 cm) at segment 8, equally enhancing in arterial phase (b). Contrast-enhanced helical CT in arterial phase (c) confirms the CEUS findings

fast scans and patients' collaboration. If these needs are adequately met, CEUS can currently also be employed to achieve reliable detection and staging of HCC.

In our previously reported experience (Solbiati 2001), a group of 48 patients with cirrhosis or chronic hepatitis (mostly HCV related) were enrolled according to the presence of at least one (even questionable) focal lesion detected with conventional sonography and elevated serum levels of alpha-fetoprotein (AFP), serum glutamic oxaloacetic transaminase (SGOT) and serum glutamic pyruvic transaminase (SGPT). A total of 80 focal lesions were

ultimately detected by means of contrast-enhanced helical CT (performed in all patients) and fine-needle aspiration biopsy (in 8 lesions), with final diagnoses of hepatocellular carcinoma (69 lesions), regenerative or dysplastic nodule (8) and hemangioma (3).

In 39 of 48 (81%) patients complete sweeps of the entire liver were technically feasible. In the remaining cases, only partial sweeps of limited areas of the liver were achievable, mostly due to insufficient inspiratory movements of patients, obesity or intrathoracic location of the liver dome. In these circumstances, a second bolus of contrast had to be

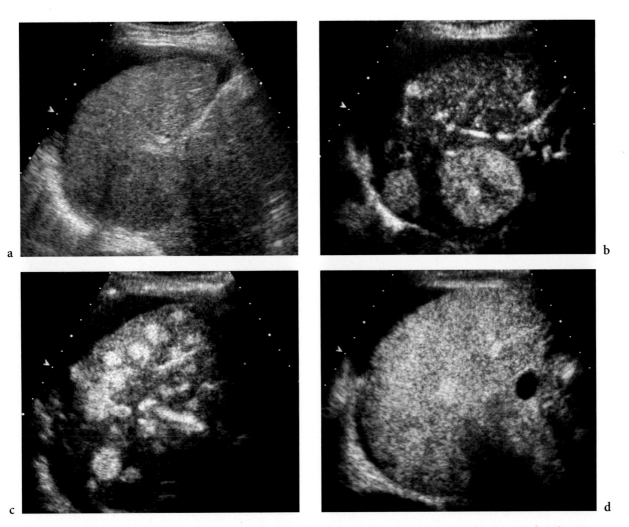

Fig. 4.42 a-d. 64-year-old patient with history of HCV-related cirrhosis and recent onset of ascites. On baseline US, a questionable mass at segment 1 is suspected (**a**). Liver echotexture is severely inhomogeneous due to diffuse fibrotic changes. On CEUS, in arterial phase, the large HCC at segment 1 is confirmed (**b**), but multiple foci of HCC undetectable on baseline US are seen in both liver lobes (**b, c**). In early portal phase, the neoplastic foci quickly washing-out become indistinguishable from the surrounding enhancing liver parenchyma (**d**)

administered in order to focus on the previously unstudied segments. Contrast-enhanced harmonic US detected 61 of the 69 HCCs seen with helical CT (Fig. 4.42), with the same conspicuity of CT (58 HCCs vs. 58 HCCs) for all but 3 patients where only 3/11 HCCs visualized by CT were detected by CEUS, mostly due to the inherent limitations of US (obesity, peculiar anatomical location of the liver, technical difficulty to perform panoramic scans of the entire liver, etc.). The sonographically detected HCCs ranged in size from 0.7 to 4.8 cm, with 43 of 61 being smaller than 2 cm. The characteristic vascular pattern of HCCs was visualized in 54 of 61 HCCs, while in the remaining 7, inhomogeneous enhancement with CEUS was related to necrotic changes and confirmed by helical CT.

Studies based on a larger number of cases and performed in different centers are essential before making any statement about the role of CEUS for the detection of HCC compared to extremely reliable imaging modalities like contrast-enhanced helical CT and MRI (*Baron et al. 1996; Bartolozzi et al. 1999; Bluemke et al. 2000; Lim 2001; Matsuo 2001*). However, since US is the imaging modality of choice for screening patients with chronic hep-

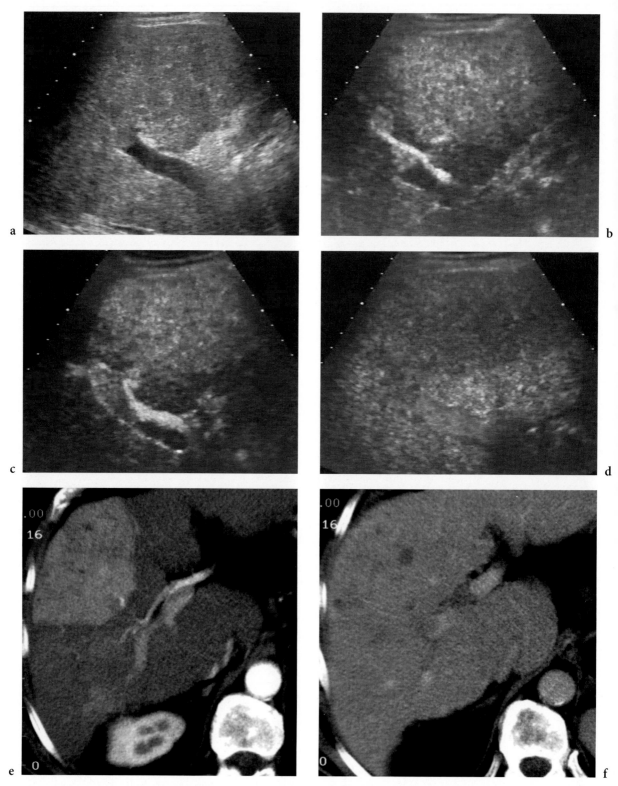

Fig. 4.43 a-f. a On baseline US, in cirrhotic liver with hepatomegaly and no evidence of focal lesions, a portal thrombus is seen at the bifurcation of the main intrahepatic portal trunk. On CEUS, at 15-20 s after contrast administration, there is early enhancement of the malignant thrombus and of a large mass at segment 8 (**b, c**). In portal phase, both the thrombus and the mass become hypoechoic (**d**). Contrast-enhanced helical CT confirms the 6-cm HCC of segment 8 in arterial phase (**e**) and the malignant portal thrombus in venous phase (**f**)

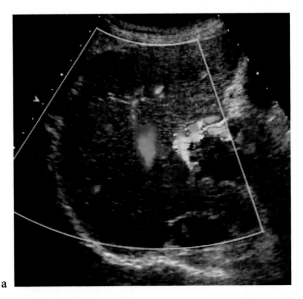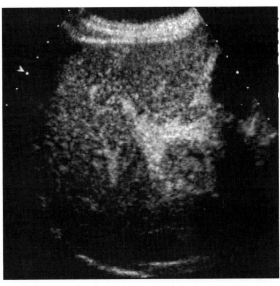

a   b

Fig. 4.44 a,b. Bland thrombus of the intrahepatic main portal trunk in liver cirrhosis. On color Doppler, blood flow signals are detected only distally to the thrombus (**a**). On CEUS, in late arterial phase, no enhancement of the thrombus is seen (**b**)

atitis and cirrhosis, CEUS with second-generation microbubbles can be suggested as an immediate second-step examination when one or more focal liver lesions are detected with baseline US, when there is discrepancy between clinical findings and US patterns, and/or when baseline US is technically poor or questionable.

An additional field of use for CEUS is the differentiation between neoplastic and bland portal venous thrombi. In more than 90% of cases, intraportal malignant thrombi enhance in the very early arterial phase, usually a few seconds before the start of the arterial enhancement of the main portion of the HCC (Fig. 4.43). On the contrary, bland thrombi do not show any contrast enhancement (Fig. 4.44).

In our experience, for the diagnosis of portal malignant thrombi, CEUS allows a significant increase in sensitivity over unenhanced color- or powerDoppler and furthermore it is not affected by motion artifacts. Thanks to the advantages of real-time study, the sensitivity of CEUS may even overcome that of contrast-enhanced helical CT or dynamic MRI.

References

Baron RL, Oliver JH 3rd, Dodd GD 3rd, Nalesnik M, Holbert BL, Carr B (1996) Hepatocellular carcinoma: evaluation with biphasic, contrast-enhanced, helical CT. Radiology 199:505-511

Bartolozzi C, Lencioni R, Donati F, Cioni D (1999) Abdominal MR: liver and pancreas. Eur Radiol 9:1496-1512

Bertolotto M, Dalla Palma L, Quaia E, Locatelli M (2000) Characterization of unifocal liver lesions with pulse inversion harmonic imaging after Levovist injection: preliminary results. Eur Radiol 10:1369-1376

Blomley MJK, Sidhu PS, Cosgrove DO, et al (2001) Do different types of liver lesions differ in their uptake of the microbubble contrast agent SHU 508A in the late liver phase ? Early experience. Radiology 220:661-667

Bluemke DA, Paulson EK, Choti MA, De Sena S, Clavien PA (2000) Detection of hepatic lesions in candidates for surgery: comparison of ferumoxides-enhanced MR imaging and dual-phase helical CT. AJR 175:1653-1658

Bruix J, Sherma M, Llovet JM, et al (2001) Clinical management of hepatocellular carcinoma. Conclusions of the Barcelona 2000 EASL Conference. J Hepatol 35:421-430

Choi BI, Park JH, Kim BH, Kim SH, Han MC, Kim CW (1989) Small hepatocellular carcinoma : detection with sonography, computed tomography (CT), angiography and lipiodol-CT. Br J Radiol 62:897-903

Choi BI, Kim AY, Lee JY, et al (2002) Hepatocellular carcinoma. Contrast enhancement with Levovist. J Ultrasound Med 21:77-84

Dill-Macky MJ, Burns PN, Khalili K, Wilson SR (2002) Focal hepatic masses: enhancement patterns with SHU 508A and pulse-inversion US. Radiology 222: 95-102

Efremidis SC, Hytiroglou P (2002) The multistep process of hepatocarcinogenesis in cirrhosis with imaging correlation. Eur Radiol 12:753-764

Kojiro M, Nakashima O. (1999) Histopathologic evaluation of hepatocellular carcinoma with special reference to small early stage tumors. Semin Liver Dis 19:287-296

Kudo M. (1999) Imaging diagnosis of hepatocellular carcinoma and premalignant/borderline lesions. Semin Liver Dis. 19:297-306

Leen E (2001) The role of contrast-enhanced ultrasound in the characterization of focal liver lesions. Eur Radiol; 11[Suppl 3]:E27-E34

Lim JH, Choi D, Cho SK, et al (2001) Conspicuity of hepatocellular nodular lesions in cirrhotic livers at ferumoxides-enhanced MR imaging: importance of Kupffer cell numbers. Radiology 220:669-676

Matsui O, Itai Y (1992). Diagnosis of primary liver cancer by computed tomography. In: Tobe T, Kameda H, Okudaira M et al, (eds) Primary liver cancer in Japan. Springer-Verlag, Tokyo, pp 132-147

Matsuo M, Kanematsu M, Itoh K, et al (2001) Detection of malignant hepatic tumors: comparison of gadolinium and ferumoxides-enhanced MR imaging. AJR 177:637-643

Numata K, Tanaka K, Kiba T, et al (2001) Contrast-enhanced, wide-band harmonic gray-scale imaging of hepatocellular carcinoma. J Ultrasound Med 20:89-98

Solbiati L, Cova L, Ierace T, Marelli P, Osti V, Goldberg SN (2000) The importance of arterial phase imaging for wideband harmonic sonography for the characterization of focal lesions in liver cirrhosis using a second generation contrast agent. Radiology 217:305

Solbiati L, Tonolini M, Cova L, Goldberg SN (2001) The role of contrast-enhanced ultrasound in the detection of focal liver lesions. Eur Radiol 11[Suppl 3]: E15-E26

Tanaka S, Ioka T, Oshikawa O, Hamada Y, Yoshioka F (2001) Dynamic sonography of hepatic tumors. AJR 177:799-805

Wilson SR, Burns PN, Murdali D, et al (2000) Harmonic hepatic US with microbubbles contrast agent: initial experience showing improved characterisation of haemangioma, hepatocellular carcinoma and metastasis. Radiology 215:147-151

4.7
Liver Metastases

A. Martegani, L. Aiani

4.7.1
Anatomical and Structural Features

Metastatic disease is by far the most frequent type of malignant focal hepatic neoplasm and the liver is the most common site for secondary tumors. Numerous types of cancer have the potential to cause hepatic metastases, but gastrointestinal and colon cancers are the most likely to spread to the liver.

Both hepatic lobes may be involved and multifocal disease is extremely frequent.

The size of the metastases can range from a few millimeters to several centimeters, depending on the nature of the primary tumor. In the case of gastrointestinal cancers, metastatic liver tumors larger than 10 cm are relatively common.

From a structural point of view, the vast majority of metastases are composed of solid nodular deposits (Fig. 4.45).

Liver metastases from ovarian cancer or certain neuroendocrine tumors can appear partially or completely cystic (Fig. 4.46).

Even when tumors appear cystic, however, there are signs of wall thickening or nodules that are not found in the case of simple cysts.

Necrotic areas are extremely common in lesions larger than 3 cm, and particularly in metastases from gastrointestinal tract primary lesions. Calcification is a frequent finding in the case of secondary lesions from mucin-secreting tumors, such as adenocarcinoma.

All metastases reveal neoangiogenic phenomena to some degree.

These new blood vessels demonstrate structural alterations of the baseline membrane (which is absent) and often show also signs of microfistula formation.

Liver metastases have microvessels within the tumor. Macrovessels are rare within the tumor but are commonly found at the periphery of the lesion. The tumor's blood supply comes mainly, but not exclusively, from arterial circulation with little or no portal contributions.

All metastases have a hematic perfusion inferior to that of the surrounding healthy parenchyma, although some tumor families (i.e., neuroendocrine, thyroid and kidney tumors) have a strong arterial inflow superior to that of the surrounding parenchyma.

Vascularization generally appears to be more conspicuous in smaller lesions (< 2 cm), with no signs of massive necrosis.

A similar vascular pattern occurs in the rare liver metastases from lymphoma or plasmocytoma.

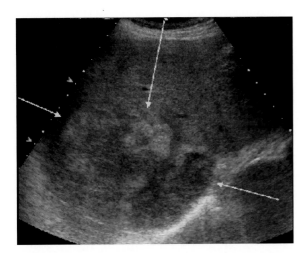

Fig. 4.45. Metastases from colon cancer. Solid, nodular, heterogeneous focal lesions with hyper-and hypoechogenic features

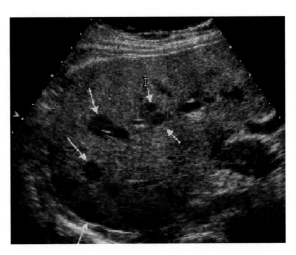

Fig. 4.46. Metastases from a neuroendocrine neoplasm: small, distinctly hypoechogenic deposits with a partially cystic component

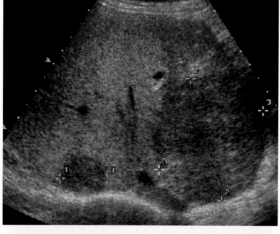
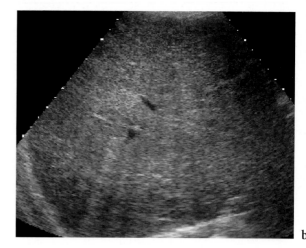
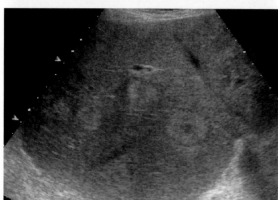

Fig. 4.47 a-c. Secondary deposits reveal a variable echogenicity, depending on the degree of hydration, cellularity, necrosis and calcification. **a** Hypoechogenic metastases from breast cancer. **b** Iso echogenic metastases from pulmonary microcytoma. **c** Hyperechogenic metastases from gastric cancer

4.7.2
Diagnostic Imaging

Ultrasound is the imaging technique most often used to study liver metastases especially in Europe.

Metastases can appear as hypo-, iso- or hyperechogenic solid nodules (Fig 4.47), depending on the origin of the primary tumor and on the presence of necrosis or calcification. In general, smaller lesions are hypo- or isoechogenic (*Brunetton et al. 1996; Cosgrove 1999; Lin et al. 1997; Harvey and Albrecht 2001*).

The larger lesions have a heterogeneous appearance, with hypoechogenic areas related to necrosis. Calcifications and fibroses appear as iso- or hyperechogenic.

The margins of the lesions may be either barely visible or well-defined (in the smallest lesions). The smallest lesions also may show a peripheral halo sign that has a target-like appearance (Fig. 4.48).

Completely cystic metastases can be confused with simple bile cysts, but the presence of septa and parietal nodes should lead the observer to suspect a malignant lesion.

Posterior enhancement (posterior acoustic trasmission) and conical shadows (shadowing) may be seen in strongly hypoechogenic lesions (melanoma or necrotic tumors) and in the case of calcification (adenocarcinoma).

Color and power Doppler scanning frequently show peripheral circulation of the metastases (Fig. 4.49) characterized by a low resistance to flow due to the presence of microfistulas; the presence of macrovessels within the lesion is relatively rare (*Nino-Murcia et al. 1992; Numata et al. 1997*).

The sensitivity and specificity of ultrasound in diagnosing secondary disease of the liver depends largely on the ability of the operator; ultrasound is generally inferior to computed tomography (CT) or magnetic resonance imaging (MRI) (*Hagspiel et al. 1995; Hollett et al.*

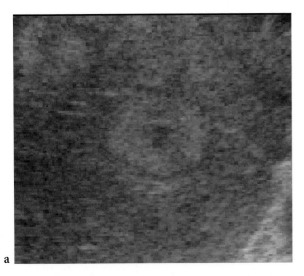

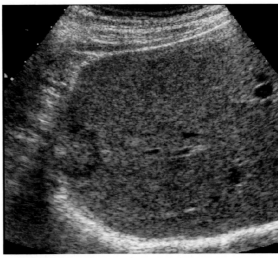

a   b

Fig. 4.48 a,b. a Target-like appearance with a thick hyperechogenic crest surrounded by a thin hypoechogenic layer. **b** Hypoechogenic ring (or halo sign) marking the periphery of the metastasis

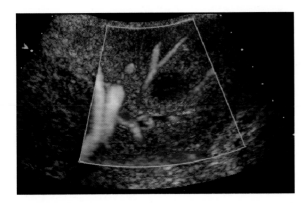

Fig. 4.49. presence of very weak vascular signals at the periphery of a small metastasis

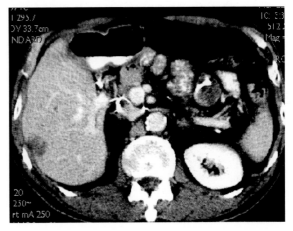

Fig. 4.50. Two metastases in the right lobe of the liver, one of them punctiform, that are easily identifiable as hypodense areas surrounded by the frankly hyperdense healthy parenchyma. The portal vessels are strongly opaque

1995; Nino-Murcia et al 2000; Van Leeunen et al. 1996; Quillin et al 1997).

Color and power Doppler, per se, do not have specific features of real clinical utility.

4.7.3
Integrated Imaging

Contrast-enhanced CT is widely used in the follow-up of secondary hepatic lesions.
The main feature of metastases is that they become less impregnated, and thus reveal lower attenuation values than the surrounding parenchyma during the portal inflow phase (more than 60 s after the injection of the contrast agent) (Fig. 4.50).

Lesions conspicuity varies according to the abundance of arterial inflow because hypervascular lesions are somewhat less visible in this phase. Therefore, supplementary scans in the late phase (at least 5 minutes after the contrast injection) are recommended.

The introduction of helical, multislice scanning equipment improved the homogenicity of

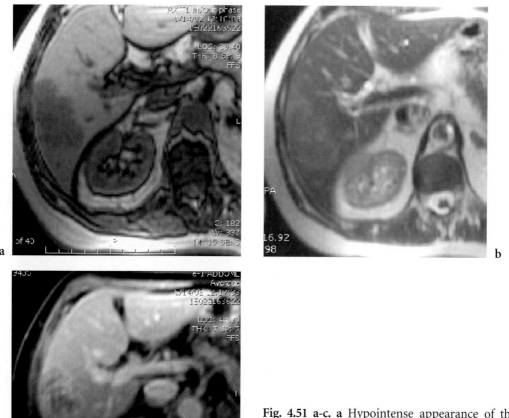

Fig. 4.51 a-c. a Hypointense appearance of the T1-weighted sequence, moderately hyperintense in the T2-dependent sequence (**b**) and target-like appearance in the portal phase after the intravenous injection of Gd BOPTA (**c**). The features of the signal in the basal sequences, combined with the signs of peripheral impregnation, are characteristic of secondary lesions

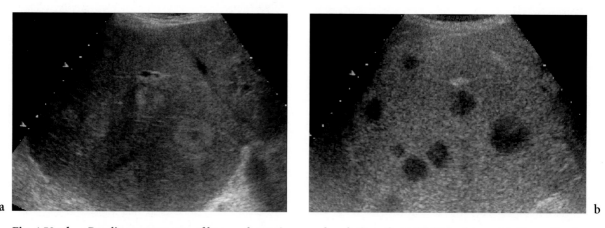

Fig. 4.52 a,b. a Baseline appearance of hyperechogenic secondary lesions. **b** At CEUS in the portal phase, the absence of any portal perfusion means that the lesions have a lower concentration of contrast medium and are therefore relatively hypoechogenic with respect to the surrounding parenchyma, which is brighter

contrast uptake throughout the liver, while reducing motion artifact.

The use of uro-angiographic paramagnetic contrast agents allows similar results with MRI (Fig. 4.51).

However, MRI also identifies lesions at baseline; metastases are generally characterized by low signal in T1-weighted sequences and a hyperintense signal in the long TR-TE sequences. Moreover, the recent introduction of contrast media with reticuloendothelial uptake and biliary elimination has improved diagnostic performance, particularly sensitivity. Currently, the utility of positron emission tomography (PET) appears to be limited by scarce spatial resolution, frequent presence of massive intralesional necrotic phenomena, and high cost.

4.7.4
Contrast-Enhanced Utrasound Imaging

The goal of CEUS is to improve the sensitivity of ultrasound detection of secondary liver disease (*Basilico et al. 2002; Bernatik et al. 2001; Blomely et al. 1999; Burns et al. 1996, 2000; Harvey et al. 2000a, 2000b; Kim et al. 2000; Leen 2002; Mattrey and Pelura 1997*).

Longer duration of clinically useful scanning times helps to achieve this goal.

Generally, the conservative technique allows an average examination time of 3–4 min, corresponding to the portal and late phases. In fact, virtually all metastases have a hypoechogenic appearance in these phases compared to the surrounding parenchyma (Fig. 4.52).

This phenomenon is determined in turn by the absence of a portal supply to the neoplastic parenchyma.

In the arterial filling phase, contrast-enhanced ultrasound (CEUS) has demonstrated that virtually all secondary lesions have an inflow that varies depending on the nature of the primary tumor and the presence of necrosis. Arterial inflow may appear particularly active in metastases from sarcomas (Fig. 4.53), neuroendocrine tumors, lymphomas or plasmocytomas (Fig. 4.54).

In other types of metastases, the arterial enhancement only partially affects the neoplastic mass due to the presence of avascular necrotic areas (Figs. 4.55, 4.56).

A peripheral ring-shaped enhancement occurs in the arterial and portal phases in 50% of metastases with a diameter of less than 3 cm (Figs. 4.57, 4.58).

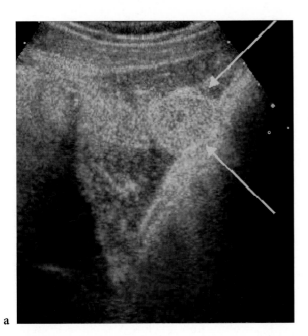 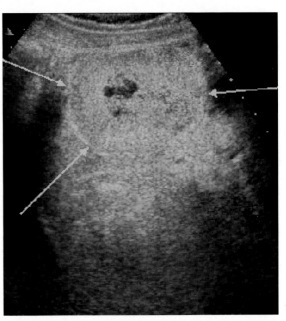

a   b

Fig. 4.53 a,b. Lively arterial impregnation of two hepatic metastases from sarcoma. The lesions are hyperechogenic because their perfusion by the contrast medium is greater than in the healthy parenchyma

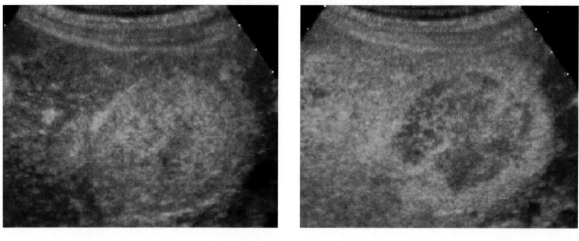

Fig. 4.54 a,b. Liver metastases from non-Hodgkin's lymphoma. In the arterial phase (**a**) there is strong impregnation by comparison with the surrounding healthy parenchyma. After 60 s, in the initial portal phase (**b**), there are signs of a marked washout and the parenchyma of the lesion becomes echogenic

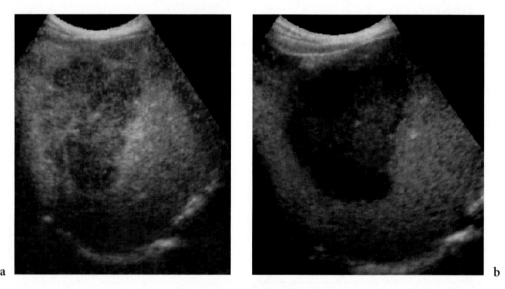

Fig. 4.55 a,b. Arterial phase (**a**) and portal phase (**b**) in metastatic disease from colorectal cancer. The arterial impregnation is irregular and heterogeneous, but easily appreciable by comparison with the image of the same lesion in the portal phase, after washout

The more conspicuous enhancement of the surrounding healthy parenchyma in the arterial phase is probably due to the presence of microfistulas that characterize the newly formed circulation. The presence of microfistulas and the increase in arterial flow due to the neoplastic microembolism of the portal sinusoids (with reduction in portal inflow and proportional increase in arterial inflow) explain the perimetastatic arterial enhancement occasionally detected in the hepatic parenchyma adjacent to the lesion.

Fast washout (within 90–120 s of the injection) is characteristic of metastases. They appear hypoechogenic and easily distinguishable from the surrounding parenchyma.

This feature is even more pronounced in lymphomatous lesions. In the late phase, the metastases are obviously hypovascular and hypoechogenic compared to the healthy liver (Fig. 4.59).

The combination of low-MI color-Doppler with B-mode imaging in the arterial phase shows scarcity of macrovessels compared to the microvascular enhancement (Fig. 4.60).

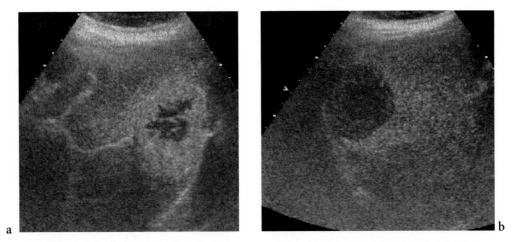

Fig. 4.56 a,b. Arterial phase (**a**) and late phase (**b**). Central avascular necrosis. The vital portion of the lesion is clearly evident in the arterial phase, but indistinguishable from the necrosis in the late phase

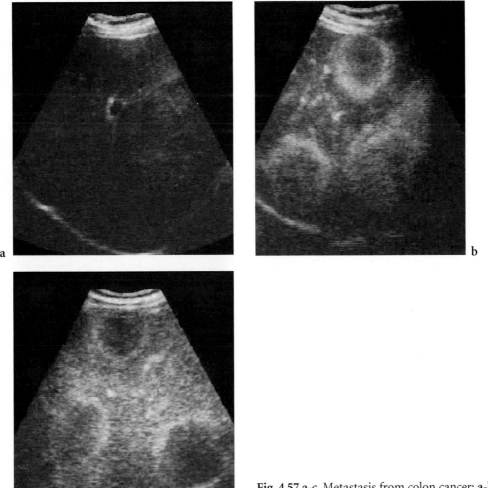

Fig. 4.57 a-c. Metastasis from colon cancer: **a**-baseline; **b**-arterial phase; **c**-portal phase. Even ring-shaped peripheral enhancement in the arterial phase. In the portal phase, the ring is still visible but less clearly

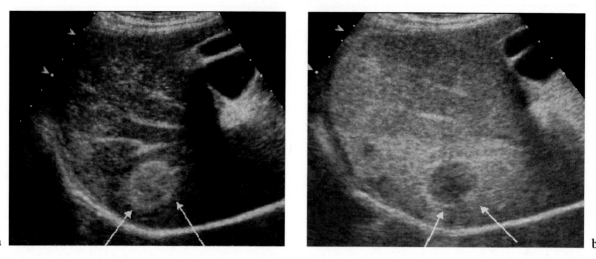

Fig. 4.58 a,b. Arterial phase (**a**) and portal phase (**b**). In this case of gastric cancer secondaries, the peripheral ring is distinctly more evident in the portal phase

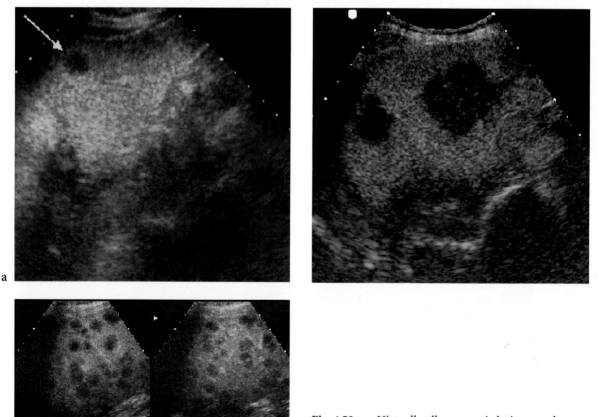

Fig. 4.59 a-c. Virtually all metastatic lesions are hypoechogenic with respect to the healthy parenchyma in the portal phase, and especially in the late phase, regardless of the tumor's organ of origin

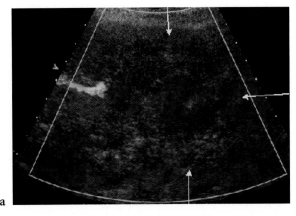
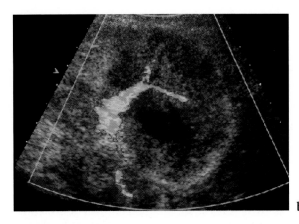

a　　　　　　　　　　　　　　　　　　　　　　　　　　　　　　　　b

Fig. 4.60 a,b. Baseline (**a**) and arterial phase (**b**). Note the scarcity of macrovascular structures within the secondary lesion. Moreover, even where impregnation is evident in the B/W image, especially at peripheral crest level, no macrovessels are apparent

Based on flow features, metastases may be characterized by:

1. Constant arterial inflow
2. Heterogeneous arterial inflow in the majority of cases
3. Rapid washout
4. Constant hypovascularity in the late phase

4.7.5
Differential Diagnostic Problems

Diffferential diagnosis may be difficult for metastatic lesions with a mainly cystic component (ovarian cancer). Parietal septa and nodules are more frequent in metastases.

Thrombosed hemangiomas may mimic the hypovascular behavior of metastases in the portal phase; however, at least a few weak vascular signals can always be identified, whereas they are entirely lacking in this type of angioma.

In patients with cirrhosis, dysplastic nodules with a markedly reduced portal inflow may mimic the behavior of secondary lesions, at least in the portal phase. In this case, signs of arterial vascularization must be sought, which are generally stronger in metastatic disease.

References

Basilico R, Blomley MJ, Harvey CJ, Filippone A, Heckemann RA, Eckersley RJ, Cosgrove DO (2002) Which continuous US scanning mode is optimal for the detection of vascularity in liver lesions when enhanced with a second generation contrast agent? Eur J Radiol 41:184-191

Bernatik T, Strobel D, Hahn EG, Becker D (2001) Detection of liver metastases: comparison of contrast-enhanced wide-band harmonic imaging with conventional ultrasonography. Ultrasound Med 20:509-515

Blomely MJK, Albrecht T, Cosgrove DO (1999) Improved imaging of liver metastases with stimulated acoustic emission in the late phase of enhancement with US contrast agent SHU 563 A; early experience. Radiology 210:409-416

Brunetton JN, Raffelli C, Balu-Maestro C, et al (1996) Sonographic diagnosis of solitary solid liver nodules in cancer patients. Eur Radiol 6:439-442

Burns PN, Powers JE, Simpson DH, et al (1996) Harmonic imaging with ultrasound contrast agents. Clin Radiol 51 [Suppl 1]:50-55

Burns PN ,Wilson SR, MD, Simpson DH (2000) Pulse inversion imaging of liver blood flow: improved method for characterizing focal masses with microbubble contrast. Invest Radiol 35:58-71

Cosgrove DO, Bolondi L (1999) Malignant liver disease. In: Cosgrove DO (ed) Abdominal and general ultrasound. Churchill Livingstone, New York, pp 271-293

Hagspiel KD, Neidl KFW, Eichenberger AC, et al. (1995) Detection of liver metastases: comparison of superparamagnetic iron oxide-enhanced and unenhanced MR imaging at 1,5 T with dynamic CT, intraoperative US, and percutaneous US. Radiology 196:471-478

Harvey CJ, Blomely MJK, Eckersley H, et al (2000a) Hepatic malignancies: improved detection with pulse inversion US in late phase with SHU 508 A; early experience. Radiology 216:903-908

Harvey CJ et al (2000b) Pulse inversion mode imaging of liver specific microbubbles. Improved detection of subcentimeters metastases. Lancet 335

Harvey CJ Albrecht T (2001) Ultrasound of focal liver lesions. Eur Radiol 11:1578-1593

Hollett MD, Jeffrey RB, Nino-Murcia M et al (1995) Dual-phase helical CT of the liver: value of arterial phase scans in the detection of small (less than 1.5 cm) malignant hepatic neoplasms AJR 164:879-884

Kim TK, Choi BI, Hong HS, et al (2000) Improved imaging of hepatic metastases with delayed pulse inversion harmonic imaging using a contrast agent SH U 508A: preliminary study. Ultrasound Med Biol 26:1439-1444

Leen E, Angerson WJ, Yarmenitis S, Bongartz G, Blomley M, Del Maschio A, Summaria V, Maresca G, Pezzoli C, Llull JB (2002) Multi-centre clinical study evaluating the efficacy of SonoVue (BR1), a new ultrasound contrast agent in Doppler investigation of focal hepatic lesions. Eur J Radiol 41:200-206

Lin ZY, Wang LY, Wang JH, et al (1997) Clinical utility of color Doppler sonography in the differentiation of hepatocellular carcinoma from metastases and hemangioma. J Ultrasound Med 16:51-58

Mattrey RF, Pelura TJ (1997) Perfluorocarbon-based ultrasound contrast agents. In: Goldberg BB (ed) Ultrasound contrast agents. Martin Dunits, pp 83-87

Nino-Murcia M, Ralls PW,Jeffrey RB Jr, et al (1992) Color Doppler characterization of focal hepatic lesions. AJR 159:1195-1197

Nino-Murcia M, Olcott EW, Jeffrey RB Jr, et al (2000) Focal liver lesions: pattern-based classification scheme for enhancement at arterial phase CT. Radiology 215:746-751

Numata K, Tanaka K, Kiba T, et al (1997) Use of hepatic tumor index on color Doppler sonography for differentiating large hepatic tumors. AJR 168: 991-995

Van Leeuwen MS, Noordzij J, Feldberg MAM, et al (1996) Focal liver lesions: characterization with triphasic spiral CT. Radiology 201:327-336

Quillin SP, Atilla S, Brown JJ, et al (1997) Characterization of focal hepatic masses by dynamic contrast-enhanced MR imaging: findings in 311 lesions. Magn Reson Imaging 15:275-285

4.8
Other Malignancies
M. Tonolini, L. Cova, V. Osti, L. Solbiati

4.8.1
Peripheral Cholangiocarcinoma

Cholangiocellular carcinoma is a malignant tumor originating from the bile duct epithelium and accounts for 10% of primary liver malignancies. According to the site of origin, it may be classified as intrahepatic or extrahepatic, the latter being more appropriately termed "bile duct carcinoma" (*Bartolozzi 2001*).

Peripheral cholangiocarcinoma arises from small intrahepatic bile duct branches. Predisposing factors include primary sclerosing cholangitis, ulcerative colitis, anomalies of the bile tract, *Clonorchis sinensis* infestation, intrahepatic stones and Thorotrast exposure (*Ros 2001*). The relationship between hepatolithiasis and cancer is not well understood: bile stasis and repeated ascending cholangitis probably lead to the development of periductal inflammation, hyperplasia and carcinoma. This neoplasm usually occurs in advanced age and the clinical picture includes ill-defined upper abdominal discomfort, anorexia and weight loss, and possibly gastrointestinal symptoms. Serum carcinoembrionic antigen (CEA) levels are raised. Late diagnosis is common, since jaundice is only present in extrahepatic bile duct tumors or in end-stage intrahepatic cholangiocarcinoma.

On gross pathology, cholangiocarcinoma may consist of multiple confluent nodules or of a large mass with lobulated contours and absence of a capsule. Tumor growth usually leads to obstruction of intrahepatic bile ducts and invasion of portal vein branches. Histology reveals a glandular adenocarcinoma with extensive intralesional fibrosis: microscopic differentiation from metastatic adenocarcinoma may be challenging (*Ros 2001*).

With conventional unenhanced ultrasound cholangiocarcinoma appears as a space-occupying solid lesion of variable size, usually located in the posterior segments of the liver. Small lesions are hypo- to isoechoic to the surrounding parenchyma (Fig. 4.61, 4,62), whereas larger lesions are mixed/hyperechoic (Fig. 4.62a). Ab-

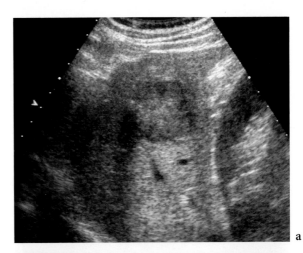

a

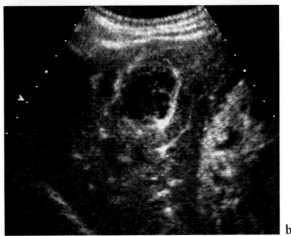

b

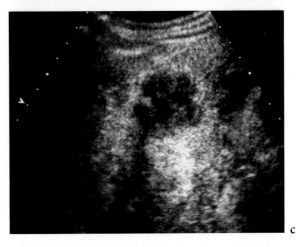

c

Fig. 4.61 a-c. 3.5-cm peripheral cholangiocellular carcinoma at segment 4, studied with baseline US (**a**) and CEUS in arterial (**b**) and portal (at 120 s) phases (**c**)

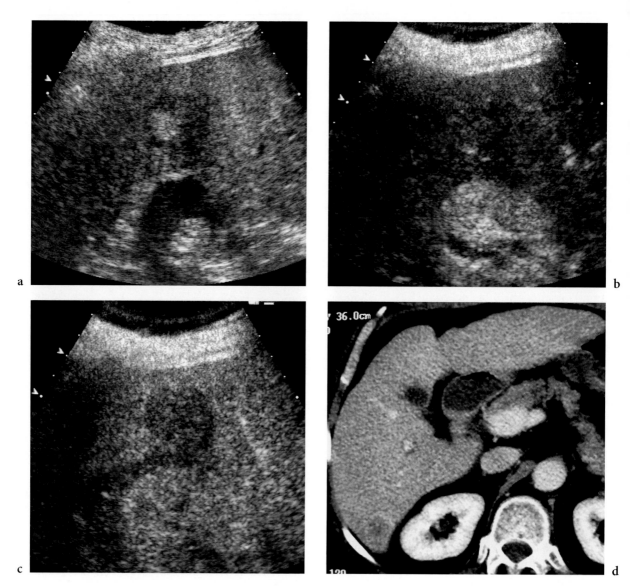

Fig. 4.62 a-d. Cholangiocellular carcinoma at segment 6, studied with baseline US (**a**). The mass is slightly hyperechoic in the middle. With CEUS, in arterial phase the lesion does not enhance (**b**), while in portal phase the tumor is clearly visualized (**c**) due to its marked hypoechogenicity compared to the surrounding liver tissue. Contrast-enhanced CT confirms the hypoenhancing pattern of the lesion (**d**), with a perilesional thin and partially enhancing halo

sence of intralesional flow signals on color Doppler reflects their hypovascularity. Peripheral bile duct dilatation – above the level of the tumor – and portal venous encasement may be visible (*Harvey and Albrecht 2001*).

On unenhanced computed tomography (CT) intrahepatic cholangiocarcinoma is a solitary, non encapsulated hypodense mass lesion with irregular margins and sometimes internal calcifications. On magnetic resonance imaging (MRI) the tumor is usually hy-

pointense on T1-weighted images and variably hyperintense on T2-weighted images according to fibrous content. Reduced T2 signal intensity corresponds to extensive intralesional fibrosis or necrotic changes. Capsular retraction, intrahepatic bile duct dilatation and vascular encasement are characteristic features (*Bartolozzi 2001*).

Contrast-enhanced sonography in arterial phase shows either complete lack of enhancement (Fig. 4.62b) or only increased echogenicity of the perilesional arterial branches supplying the mass (Fig. 4.61b). In early portal phase, cholangiocarcinomas are likely to be indistinguishable from the surrounding normal liver parenchyma, while the most characteristic feature is the progressively decreasing echogenicity compared to liver tissue in full and delayed portal phases (Figs. 4.61c, 4.62c). The best visualization of the tumor is usually achieved at 120-180 s after contrast bolus administration.

These features shown by contrast-enhanced ultrasound (CEUS) strictly correspond to the findings achievable with contrast-enhanced CT and MRI, which mostly demonstrate minimal to moderate, thin and incomplete peripheral enhancement (Fig. 4.62d). However, in a minority of cases, CT and MRI may show some progressive centripetal fill-in in portal phase, with persistent although heterogeneous enhancement ("pooling of contrast" due to fibrous stroma) in the delayed phase (*Bartolozzi 2001*). The possibility of achieving also this type of enhancement with CEUS has not been reported yet, probably due to the very small number of cholangiocarcinomas reportedly studied with CEUS and second-generation contrast agents so far.

4.8.2
Hepatic Sarcoma

Angiosarcoma is a malignant neoplasm that originates from the endothelium and is the most frequent mesenchymal liver malignancy in adult patients (*Bartolozzi 2001*). Exposure to Thorotrast, vinyl chloride and inorganic arsenic represent causative factors. This very rare tumor is predominantly diagnosed in men between the sixth and eighth decade of life, and its presence may be revealed by intraperitoneal hemorrhage or by hepatic failure. The clinical course is highly aggressive with metastases to the lungs and an extremely poor prognosis (*Ros 2001*).
Other even less common sarcomas of the liver include leiomyosarcoma, malignant fibrous histiocytoma and fibrosarcoma. Also these types of malignancies are more frequent in adults and elderly patients.

All these malignancies often reach large size before detection with imaging modalities. They are usually located at the liver surface and have two different growth patterns: large unencapsulated solitary mass or multifocal nodules (ranging in size from millimetric foci to several centimeters; Fig. 4.63a) (*Ros 2001*).

Conventional ultrasound depicts sarcomas as medium- to large-sized masses of mixed echogenicity due to hemorrhagic or necrotic changes. Color Doppler may detect the presence of some intralesional flow signals. CEUS shows persistent hypoenhancement compared to liver tissue in all the vascular phases (Fig. 4.63b,c)

Unenhanced CT demonstrates sarcomas as nonspecific low-attenuation lesions. Hyperdense areas may be observed if fresh hemorrhage or Thorotrast deposits are present (*Ros 2001*).

On MRI these tumors are strongly hyperintense on T2-weighted images since they contain abundant blood-filled spaces. On contrast-enhanced studies, peripheral, usually heterogeneous enhancement is observed and lesions appear hypovascular on postcontrast images (*Bartolozzi 2001*).

4.8.3
Hepatic Lymphoma

Primary hepatic lymphoma is diagnosed when the involvement is limited to the hepatic parenchyma and is a rare occurrence. Hepatic involvement is possible in the course of both Hodgkin's and non-Hodgkin's systemic lymphomas, and has recently been increasingly seen in patients with AIDS and in post-transplantation lymphoproliferative disorders. Hodgkin's disease involves the liver in the form of miliary deposits, and nodular-type lesions may develop over time. Conversely, most types of non-Hodgkin's lymphomas form nodular masses. The periportal area is most commonly involved since it is the richest area of lymphatic tissue in the liver (*Bartolozzi 2001*).

On conventional US, hepatic lymphomatous lesions appear as hypoechoic nodules or masses (Fig. 4.64a), sometimes cyst-like. In the diffuse form, the level of echogenicity of liver parenchyma is normal, but its architecture is diffusely altered.

Lymphomatous nodules demonstrate decreased attenuation values on unenhanced CT

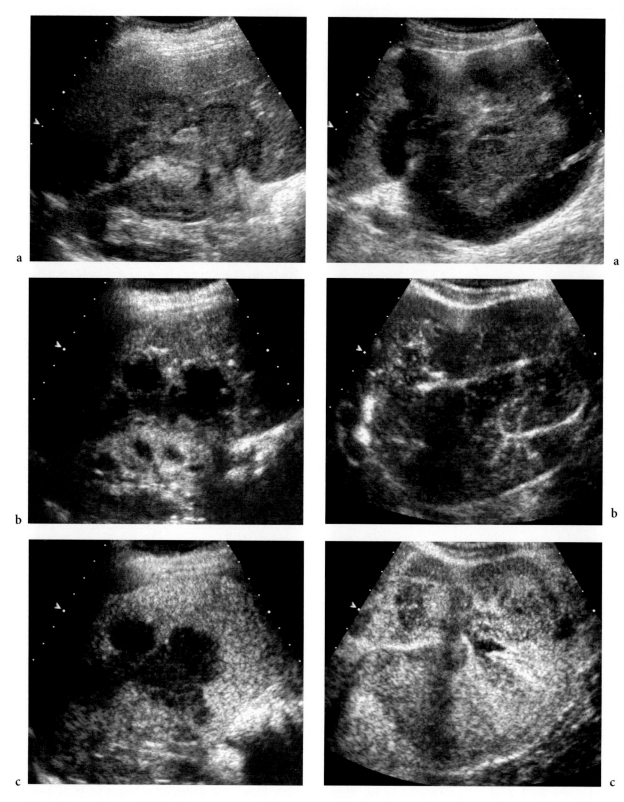

Fig. 4.63 a-c. Large, multinodular leiomyosarcoma at segment 6, close to the hepatorenal space, studied with baseline US (**a**). After contrast bolus injection, CEUS shows persistent hypoechogenicity of the tumor both in arterial (**b**) and in portal phases (**c**)

Fig. 4.64 a-c. Large Hodgkin lymphomatous mass at segments 5 and 6, studied with baseline US (**a**) and CEUS, with typical hypovascularity in both vascular phases (arterial in **b** and portal in **c**)

scans and are T1-hypointense and T2-hyperintense on MRI due to the rich cellularity (*Bartolozzi 2001*).

On CEUS, in the arterial phase the major arteries supplying the mass clearly enhance (Fig. 4.64b), but the tumor microvascularity does not enhance due to the predominant hypercellularity of these malignancies. In portal phase, the enhancement is slower, less intense and more inhomogeneous than that of liver parenchyma (Fig. 4.64c).

On dynamic contrast-enhanced studies with CT and MRI, too, lymphomatous masses remain permanently hypodense or hypointense during all the vascular phases, owing to their poor vascularity (*Bartolozzi 2001*).

References

Bartolozzi C, Cioni D, Donati F, Lencioni R (2001) Focal liver lesions: MR imaging-pathologic correlation. Eur Radiol 11:1374-1388

Harvey CJ, Albrecht T (2001). Ultrasound of focal liver lesions. Eur Radiol 11:2578-2593

Ros PR, Menu Y, Vilgrain V, Mortele KJ, Terris B (2001) Liver neoplasms and tumor-like conditions. Eur Radiol 11 [Suppl 2] S145-S165

5 Medical Needs

E. Leen

5.1
Introduction

Due its relative low cost, safety and availability, conventional ultrasound (US) remains the most widely used cross-sectional imaging modality in routine clinical practice worldwide. Recent advances in nonlinear imaging together with a whole new generation of echo-enhancing agents have improved the clinical applications of US. Indeed there are now increasing reports of single- and multicenter studies confirming improved detection and characterization of focal liver lesions with contrast-enhanced US (*Albrecht et al. 2001; Bernatik et al. 2001; Needleman et al. 2000; Wilson et al. 2000; Leen et al. 2002a*). In a study comparing unenhanced versus contrast-enhanced US in the detection of liver metastases, the average number of confirmed metastases increased from 3.06 to 5.42 following contrast administration; the sensitivity for detecting individual metastases significantly improved from 63% to 91%. More importantly subcentimeter lesions were identified in over 92% of confirmed cases following contrast compared with 54% at baseline (*Albrecht et al. 2001*). In a multicenter study of 123 patients evaluating unenhanced versus contrast-enhanced US in the detection of liver metastases, similar results were observed with the sensitivity for detection of individual lesions improving significantly from 71% to 87% following contrast administration. Furthermore, the specificity also improved significantly from 60% to 88% (*Albrecht et al. 2002*). In a more recent multicenter study of 157 patients, off-site blinded readers showed improved sensitivity

for detection of individual lesions from 38% to 67% following contrast injection, and the characterization of the lesions was also improved with none of the metastases showing contrast uptake in the late phase (*Leen et al. 2002b*). However, all the above studies used contrast enhanced dual-phase computed tomography (CT) and magnetic resonance imaging (MRI) scans as the standard of reference and it remains to be seen whether contrast-enhanced US is as sensitive or more accurate than CT or MRI.

Despite the significant improvement of contrast-enhanced US in imaging the liver, there is some debate as to its implementation in routine clinical practice. Clearly it is highly unlikely that it would replace CT or MRI; however, it should be used as a complementary tool in specific clinical scenarios, which are reviewed in this article.

5.2
Incidental Lesions in Normal Livers

Benign hepatic tumors or tumor-like conditions occur more frequently than anticipated in the general population. In a consecutive necropsy study of 95 men, benign lesions were identified in 52% of the cases (*Karhunen 1986*). The commonest tumors were small bile duct tumors followed by cavernous hemangiomas detected in 26 (27%) and 19 (20%) men, respectively. Multiple lesions were present in 46% of the bile duct tumors and in 50% of the hemangiomas. In another autopsy series of 95 men, half of whom had a history of alcohol abuse, preneoplastic nodules (hyperplastic and dysplastic nodules) were identified in 19% of the cases (*Karhunen and Penttila 1987*).

Small hepatic lesions are indeed frequently detected on routine imaging studies. In a contrast-enhanced abdominal CT scan review of 1,454 patients, Jones and colleagues reported the presence of hepatic lesions measuring 15 mm or less in 254 (17%) patients (1992). Of these, 130 (51%) were judged to be benign, 56 (22%) were judged to be malignant and the remaining 68 (27%) could not be classified. Eighty-two per cent of the patients with small lesions were also known to have a malignant primary tumor and in 51% of these patients, the lesions were classified as benign. None of the patients without a known malignant primary cancer had a small hepatic lesion that was classified as malignant. Multiple small hepatic lesions were more likely to represent malignancy than solitary small lesions.

More recently, in a CT report review of 2,978 patients with cancer, small lesions measuring 1 cm or less were identified in 378 (12.7%) patients (*Schwartz et al. 1999*); of these patients, the small lesions were classified as being metastases in 59 (15.6%) cases. In contrast, in 303 (80.2%) patients, the lesions were judged to be benign and in the remaining patients, the lesions were judged as indeterminate. Among the three most common primary tumors in the study, i.e., lymphoma, colorectal and breast, small lesions were metastases in 4%, 14% and 22%, respectively. The authors concluded that although small hepatic lesions in patients with cancer are more likely to be benign than malignant, these lesions represent metastases in 11.6% of patients.

Studies carried out by Jones et al. (1992) and Schwartz et al. (1999) used CT scanners in the nonhelical mode. Clearly more liver lesions would be detected with biphasic injection of contrast media, thinner collimation and helical CT scanning; the true incidence for small hepatic lesions is therefore underestimated.

The widespread use of new generations of imaging modalities has led to an increase in the frequency of detecting coincidental focal liver lesions in patients with no symptomatic evidence of liver disease. Differentiation between the benign and malignant lesions is usually not difficult when they are large, but when they are small, characterization is clearly problematic as they do not display enough characteristic features and biopsy can be very difficult if not impossible. In patients without known cancer, nearly all of these lesions will be benign and are now usually evaluated with serial follow-up imaging scans. However, in patients with known cancer where knowledge of stage and progression is crucial in determining prognosis and therapeutic management, the relevance of urgent accurate characterization of these small lesions is an important issue. Contrast-enhanced US may be of particular value in that respect.

5.3
Screening and Surveillance for Hepatocellular Carcinoma

Hepatocellular carcinoma is the fifth most common cancer in the world. In the Western world, the age-adjusted incidence rates range between 2.7 to 3.2 and men are more frequently affected than women (2:1 ratio; *Bosch and Ribes 2000*). There is a marked difference in the incidence of hepatocellular carcinoma throughout the world, with the highest incidence in East/South-East Asia, Japan, Africa and the Pacific Islands and the lowest incidence in northern Europe and northern America.

Screening and surveillance for hepatocellular carcinoma remains a clinical challenge. Despite the lack of concrete evidence of any true survival benefit or cost effectiveness, it is now becoming widely accepted among hepatologists that it should be routine in the management of patients with end-stage liver disease. Nevertheless some of the rationales for screening and surveillance are compelling.

The worldwide incidence is increasing but more noticeably in North America and Europe; it is now believed that the rise in these continents, which is progressively affecting younger patients, is mainly attributed to the rise in hepatitis C viral infection, whilst the rates associated with alcoholic cirrhosis and hepatitis B virus infection have remained stable (*El-Serag and Mason 2000*). The disease is extremely lethal with median survival rates of untreated symptomatic cases ranging between 4 and 6 months. Patients with even small tumors also carry a significant mortality as less than 50% will survive 5 years despite undergoing apparently curative resection.

The target population for screening and surveillance for hepatocellular carcinoma is readily identifiable. Chronic hepatitis B and C virus infections are well recognized to increase the risk of hepatocellular carcinoma. In Europe, approximately 28% of liver cancer has been attributed to chronic hepatitis B virus infection and 21% to hepatitis C virus infection (*Bosch and Ribes 2000*), but the risk is greatest in the presence of coinfection with both hepatitis B and C virus; male sex and alcohol abuse are significant risk factors (*Benvegnu et al. 1994*). Cirrhosis is another major risk factor irrespective of the etiology. The annual risk of developing hepatocellular carcinoma in cirrhosis ranges between 1% and 6% (*Colombo et al. 1991; Zoli et al. 1996*). The risk is higher in patients with cirrhosis caused by viral infection compared with nonviral causes.

However, patients with cirrhosis as a result of genetic hemochromatosis also have high rates of hepatocellular carcinoma. In a prospective study of 152 patients with hemochromatosis (homazygotes) by Fargion and colleagues (1994), 29% of those with liver cirrhosis developed hepatocellular carcinoma, whilst none of those without cirrhosis developed hepatocellular carcinoma; age over 55 years, presence of HbsAg and alcohol abuse increased the relative risk of hepatocellular carcinoma by 13.3-, 4.9- and 2.3-fold, respectively.

In contrast, the estimated incidence of hepatocellular carcinoma in patients with primary biliary cirrhosis is 2.4% (*Jones et al. 1997*). The development of hepatocellular carcinoma appears to be restricted to patients with stage-III/IV disease and the incidence is 5.9% in that category. The male sex has a significant impact on disease outcome; the incidence of hepatocellular carcinoma in female patients is low compared to male patients (4.1% vs 20%). In the presence of advanced disease the incidence

for male compared to female patients is even higher (45.4% vs 8.3%). The reason for the increased risk of hepatocellular carcinoma development in male compared to female cirrhotic patients with primary biliary cirrhosis is unclear. It has been suggested that this may be the result of increased incidence of underlying risk etiologies such as alcohol abuse and chronic hepatitis B carriage in males. However, in the study report of Jones and colleagues (1997), such confounding etiological factors including hepatitis B and C, alcoholic liver disease and hemochromatosis have been excluded, which therefore confirms that the risk for hepatocellular carcinoma is truly increased in males.

The incidence of hereditary causes of cirrhosis such as Wilson disease, alpha-1-antitrypsin deficiency, galactosemia, type-IV glycogen storage disease, tyrosinemia, Osler-Weber-Rendu syndrome and familial cirrhosis and autoimmune cirrhosis is not clearly established but is presumably much lower than the above-mentioned well-recognized etiologies.

Whilst cirrhosis is a major risk factor irrespective of etiology, up to 56% of patients presenting with hepatocellular carcinoma have previously undiagnosed cirrhosis (*Zaman et al. 1990*). Cirrhosis may be easily diagnosed by any cross-sectional imaging modality if characteristic features such as nodular hepatic contour, ascites and/or varices are present. But in the early stages of the disease, it may be impossible to differentiate between stage-III fibrosis and cirrhosis. If the presence of cirrhosis alone were to be used to define the target population, these patients would not have been recruited into the screening or surveillance program. Zaman and colleagues (1990) also showed that those patients with occult cirrhosis were predominantly HbsAg-seropositive. Therefore patients with chronic viral hepatitis as well as those with overt cirrhosis have to be included in any screening or surveillance program.

Serum alpha-fetoprotein (AFP) levels and conventional US have been the most commonly used screening tests for hepatocellular carcinoma with low morbidity. The ideal screening tests should also have high sensitivity and specificity. But the performance of AFP has been poor in that respect with a sensitivity of 39%-64%, a specificity of 76%-91% and a positive predictive value of 9%-32% (*Pateron et al. 1994; Oka et al. 1994; Sherman et al. 1995*). In addition, rise in AFP levels is not specific for hepatocellular carcinoma and it may also increase transiently, persistently or intermittently with flares of active hepatitis. In contrast, within the context of screening healthy HbsAg carriers as well as cirrhotic patients, US has been shown to have a sensitivity of 71% and 78%, respectively, a specificity of 93% but a positive predictive value of 14% and 73% respectively (*Sherman et al. 1995; Pateron et al. 1994*). These could be improved further with the administration of contrast.

Previous reported surveillance intervals ranged between 3 and 12 months and it is now generally accepted that the intervals should be 6 months taking into account the reported median tumor doubling time, which is about 117 days (*Sheu et al. 1985*).

There are as yet no studies to determine the best recall policy. However, at the consensus meeting of the European Association for the Study of Liver in Barcelona in 2000, it suggested that cirrhotic patients should undergo 6-monthly US and AFP level assessment. Patients who have no nodules on US but have increasing AFP levels should undergo spiral CT of the liver. For those patients with a nodule of less than 1 cm, 3-monthly US is recommended on the basis that these lesions are far too small to characterize accurately and at least 50% of these sub-centimeter lesions will not be hepatocellular carcinomas. Patients with a nodule of over 2 cm should have AFP levels over 400 ng/ml and CT, MRI or angiography evidence of lesional hypervascularity before hepatocellular carcinoma can be confirmed (*Bruix et al. 2001*). If the nodule is less than 2 cm, diagnosis can be made using noninvasive criteria (if biopsy is not an option) which have been defined as: (a) radiological criteria – two coincidental imaging techniques showing arterial hypervascularization for lesions over 2 cm; (b) combined criteria – one imaging modality showing arterial hypervascularization associated with AFP levels over 400 ng/ml. Biopsy may be another option in some centers, but remains controversial; in some North American

and European centers, biopsy would prelude hepatic resection or transplant because of risk of tumor seedlings along the needle tracks. Furthermore, a negative biopsy of a lesion visible on imaging in a cirrhotic liver does not necessarily rule out malignancy completely. Therefore within the context of the cirrhotic patient, hepatocellular carcinoma can be diagnosed noninvasively using the above-mentioned criteria. Accurate staging of the hepatocellular carcinoma is important in determining the optimal therapeutic management. US is widely accepted to be adequate in diagnosing advanced-stage disease with no therapeutic options; however, in planning for resection, triple-phase contrast-enhanced CT or MRI are recommended as they are the most accurate, and hepatic angiography has largely been replaced by these techniques.

Clearly there are several stages in this algorithm whereby administration of US contrast might be more effective, namely: (a) in the 6-monthly recalls to improve detection, (b) the characterization of the lesions measuring less than 2 cm and (c) as the second modality in demonstrating the hypervascularity of the lesion in the noninvasive diagnosis of hepatocellular carcinoma.

5.4
Staging and Follow-up of Cancer Patients

Accurate cancer staging is crucial in determining the optimal therapeutic management of the patients and is highly dependent upon imaging studies. The liver is the commonest target organ for metastasis for many primary cancers. There are therefore clinically distinct tasks in liver imaging, which include firstly the assessment of whether there is any tumor deposit in the liver, secondly the characterization of the lesion, and thirdly to stage the tumor in the liver for resection, i.e., to determine the extent and localization of intrahepatic disease, the involvement of surgically critical areas such as the porta hepatis and major bile ducts, and the presence of extrahepatic disease.

Imaging strategies for the liver will also differ, depending on the clinical setting. Different techniques are required depending on: (a) primary tumor types, (b) evaluation prior to resection of the primary, (c) surveillance of patients who had undergone apparently curative resection of the primary cancer, (d) follow-up examinations for patients with known liver metastases to assess therapeutic response, and (f) evaluations prior to surgical hepatic resection in which more rigorous study is required to locate all hepatic lesions. For example, a single imaging modality such as US, CT or MRI may be adequate to screen for the presence or absence of metastases or for assessment of metastasis response to treatment, but multiple imaging studies (multiphasic contrast-enhanced CT, MRI or intraoperative US) are often required when liver resection of metastases is being considered.

In many centers, hepatic US remains the primary modality of choice in imaging the liver for suspected metastases from primary tumors such as: breast, *skin*, esophagus, stomach, pancreas and lung. This practice is merely historical, readily available and cheap (compared to CT or MRI) and is usually triggered by the patient's abnormal liver function tests; the identification of liver metastasis is also simply used as a prognostic indicator of poor outcome. For these tumor types, in contrast to colorectal cancer, "global detection" of hepatic metastasis, i.e., whether metastasis is present or not, is the most important issue rather than "the actual number and localization" of the metastasis, as liver resection is usually not an option. In that respect, US sensitivity has been reported to be as high as 85% and may in fact be improved with the use of echo-enhancers (*Freeny 1988; Clarke et al. 1989*).

Intraoperative US remains the most sensitive imaging modality relative to current multiphasic contrast CT or MRI in the detection of hepatic metastasis and is routinely used prior to liver resection by most liver surgeons. CT is, however, still required to rule out any extrahepatic disease before liver resection is contemplated. It is commonly known that the 5-year survival of patients undergoing liver resection for metastases ranges between 30% and 40% at best; the majority of the patients ultimately succumb to residual disease or

"occult" metastases, which remained undetectable to conventional imaging modalities at the time of resection. It remains to be seen whether contrast-enhanced intraoperative US can identify these occult metastases, and there are studies currently underway to assess its value.

For patients who undergo apparently curative resection of the primary cancer, there are centers, which undertake a formal or semi-formal type of surveillance program for early detection of recurrence on the premise that if detected early, these patients would stand a better chance for prolonged survival or even cure. However, similar to the screening programs for hepatocellular carcinoma, there is as yet no evidence to suggest that surveillance for recurrence is cost effective or actually improves survival. Recent studies have highlighted the lack of consensus among surgeons on the value of routine follow-up after curative resection for the primary cancer, in particular colorectal cancer which is a good example given it is the second commonest cause of cancer death in the Western world (*Mella et al. 1997; Foster et al. 1987*). However, most studies have focused on the early detection of local recurrence amenable to surgery, but these are clearly based on a false premise and there is increasing evidence that this approach is ineffective and costly (*Biggs and Ballantyne 1994*). In contrast, surveillance programs designed to detect asymptomatic liver metastases may be more effective. Indeed, more recently, Howell and colleagues (1999) have shown that an intensive liver imaging follow-up program with 3-monthly US and yearly CT identified 88% of patients who developed liver metastases in an asymptomatic stage and were amenable to liver resection or chemotherapy. It is worth noting that the 5-year survival of patients undergoing liver resection is about 35% and mortality is usually less than 5% (*Ballantyne 1993*). Furthermore, recent studies have shown that patients with disseminated disease receiving systemic chemotherapy at an asymptomatic stage had higher response rates, better quality of life and improved survival compared with those in whom the administration of chemotherapy was delayed until they became symptomatic (Nordic Gastrointestinal Tumour

Adjuvant Therapy Group 1992). The question of imaging in follow-up programs and its intensity should therefore be readdressed. Although CT may be effective for detection of both local and hepatic recurrences, it is also more expensive and less readily available than US, but the latter is limited in the detection of local recurrence in routine practice. However, local recurrence usually occurs within the first 6 months of the primary resection; a follow-up program could therefore be tailored to using US beyond the first 6 months.

Contrast-enhanced US may be a more cost-effective modality in the detection of liver metastases given the constraints of current health resources.

References

Albrecht T, Hoffmann CW, Schmitz SA, et al (2001) Phase inversion sonography during the liver specific late phase of contrast enhancement: improved detection of liver metastases. AJR 176:1191-1198

Albrecht T, Blomley MKJ, Burns PN, et al (2002) Improved detection of hepatic metastases with pulse inversion ultrasonography during the liver specific phase of SHU 508A(Levovist) – a multi-centre study. Radiology (in press)

Ballantyne GH (1993) Surgical treatment of liver metastases in patients with colorectal cancer. Cancer 71:4252-4266

Benvegnu L, Fattovich G, Noventa, et al (1994) Concurrent hepatitis B and C virus infection and risk of hepatocellular carcinoma in cirrhosis. A prospective study. Cancer 74:2442-2448

Bernatik T, Strobel D, Hahn EG, Becker D (2001) Detection of liver metastases. Comparison of contrast enhanced wide band harmonic imaging with conventional ultrasonography. J Ultrasound Med 20:509-515

Biggs CG, Ballantyne GH (1994) Sensitivity versus cost effectiveness in post operative follow-up for colorectal cancer. Curr Opnion Gen Surg 94-102

Bosch FX, Ribes J (2000) Epidemiology of liver cancer in Europe. Can J Gastroenterol 14:621-30

Bruix J, Sherman M, Llovet JM, et al (2001) Clinical management of hepatocellular carcinoma. Conclusions of the Barcelona-EASL Conference. J Hepatol. 35:421-430

Clarke MR, Kane RA, Steele G Jr, et al (1989) Prospective comparison of pre-operative imaging and intraoperative ultrasonography in the detection of liver tumours. Surgery 106:849-855

Colombo M, De Franchis R, Del Ninno E, et al (1991) Hepatocellular carcinoma in Italian patients with cirrhosis. Lancet 325:675-680

El-Serag HB, Mason AC (2000) Risk factors for the rising rates of primary liver cancer in the United States. Arch Intern Med 160:3227-3230

Fargion S, Fracanzani AL, Piperno A, et al (1994) Prognostic factors for hepatocellular carcinoma in genetic haemochromatosis. Hepatology 10:1426-1431

Foster ME, Hill J, Leaper DJ (1987) Follow-up after colorectal cancer-current practice in Wales and South West England. Int J Colorectal Dis 2: 118-119

Freeny PC (1988) Hepatic CT: state of the art. Radiology 168:319-323

Howell JD, Wotherspoon H, Leen E, et al (1999) Evaluation of a follow-up programme after curative resection for colorectal cancer. Br J Cancer 79:308-310

Jones DE, Metcalf JV, Collier JD, Bassendine MF, James OF (1997) Hepatocellular carcinoma in primary biliary cirrhosis and its impact on outcomes. Hepatology 26:1138-1142

Jones EC, Chezmar JL, Nelson RC, Bernardino ME (1992) The frequency and significance of small (less than or equal 15mm) hepatic lesions detected by CT. AJR 158:535-539

Karhunen PJ (1986) Benign hepatic tumours and tumour like conditions in men. J Clin Pathol 39:183-188

Karhunen PJ, Penttila A (1987). Pre-neoplastic lesions of human liver. Hepatogastroenterology 34:10-15

Leen E, Correas JM, Needleman L, et al (2002a) Multicentre study of Sonazoid enhanced sonography of patients with known primary cancer: improved detection of liver metastases. (Abstract) Radiology (in press)

Leen E, Angerson WJ, Yarmenitis S, et al (2002b) Multicentre clinical study evaluating the efficacy of SonoVue in Doppler investigation of focal hepatic lesions. Eur J Radiol 41:200-206

Mella J, Datta SN, Biffin A, et al (1997) Surgeons follow-up practice after resection of colorectal cancer. Ann R Coll Surg England 79:206-209

Needleman L, Leen E, Kyriakopoulou K, et al (2000) NC100100, a new liver specific contrast agent for fundamental and harmonic imaging of hepatic lesions. (Abstract) Radiology 209:189

Nordic Gastrointestinal Tumour Adjuvant Therapy Group (1992) Expectancy or primary chemotherapy in patients with advanced asymptomatic colorectal cancer; a randomised trial. J Clin Oncol 10:904-911

Oka H, Tamori A, Kuroki T, Kobayashi K, Yamamoto S (1994) Prospective study of alpha-fetoprotein in cirrhotic patients monitored for development of hepatocellular carcinoma. Hepatology 19:61-66

Pateron D, Ganne N, Trinchet JC, et al (1994) Prospective study of screening for hepatocellular carcinoma in Caucasian patients with cirrhosis. J Hepatol 20:65-71

Schwartz LH, Gandras EJ, Colangelo SM, Ercolani MC, Panicek DM (1999) Prevalence and importance of small hepatic lesions found at CT in patients with cancer. Radiology 210:71-74

Sherman M, Peltekian KM, Lee C (1995) Screening for hepatocellular carcinoma in chronic carriers of hepatitis B virus: incidence and prevalence of hepatocellular carcinoma in a North American urban population. Hepatology 22:432-438

Sheu JC, Chen DS, Sung JL, et al (1985) Hepatocellular carcinoma in the early stage. Radiology 155:463-467

Wilson SR, Burns PN, Muradali D, et al (2000) Harmonic hepatic US with microbubble contrast agent: initial experience showing improved characterisation of haemangioma, hepatocellular carcinoma and metastasis. Radiology 215:153-161

Zaman SN, Johnson PJ, Williams R (1990) Silent cirrhosis in patients with hepatocellular carcinoma. Implications for screening in high incidence and low incidence areas. Cancer 65:1607-1610

Zoli M, Magalotti D, Bianchi G, Gueli C, Marchenisi G, Pisa E (1996) Efficacy of surveillance program for early detection of hepatocellular carcinoma. Cancer 78:977-985

6 Guidance and Control of Percutaneous Treatments

L. Solbiati, M. Tonolini, L. Cova

6.1
Introduction

Over the past decade, extensive changes have occurred in the therapeutic approach to primary and metastatic hepatic malignancies. Currently, percutaneous interventional modalities such as ethanol injection (PEI) and thermal ablation using different energy sources including radiofrequency (RF), laser or microwave are widely accepted for minimally invasive treatment of liver tumors (*Goldberg et al. 2000; Dodd et al. 2000*).

Among these, RF ablation is currently by far the most used technique for both hepatocellular carcinoma and liver metastases and the number of treated patients is steadily increasing. Several large series demonstrated its safety and effectiveness and pointed out its significant advantages, including feasibility in nonsurgical candidates, the possibility of repeated treatment sessions if local recurrence or new lesions develop, lower morbidity and mortality compared to surgical resection, and markedly reduced treatment costs and hospital stays (*Livraghi et al. 1999, 2000, 2001; Solbiati et al. 1997b*). The results of RF ablation compare favorably in terms of survival with those reported in recent surgical series, although patients are usually not candidates for resection (*Solbiati et al. 2001; Buscarini et al. 2001*).

6.2
Fundamentals and Pathology of Ablative Treatments

The common final goal of ablative therapies is to achieve local complete destruction of neoplastic lesions.

Ethanol injection induces cellular dehydration and protein denaturation, resulting in coagulative necrosis of the tumoral tissue. In addition, ethanol produces a chemical vasculitis followed by thrombosis of small vessels within and around the tumor. Similarly, thermal ablation modalities achieve coagulation necrosis with the application of adequately high local temperatures (above 50°C for 10–12 min) through a mechanism of protein denaturation and irreversible inactivation of cellular and mitochondrial enzymes and of nucleic acid–histone complexes. Finally, all ablative treatments lead to the disruption of tumor vascularity: the best way to noninvasively assess the efficacy of any percutaneous ablation is the demonstration of blood supply disruption inside and at the periphery of the tumor by means of imaging methods.

The main limitations of thermal ablative therapies include the possible inhomogeneity of heat deposition, a variable cytotoxicity with heating and, more importantly, the cooling effect of blood flow. In recent years technical developments that improve tissue–energy interactions, including internally cooled electrodes (*Goldberg et al. 1996*), cluster electrodes (*Goldberg et al. 1998*), pulsed current application (*Goldberg et al. 1999*) and peritumoral saline injection prior to energy deposition (*Livraghi et al. 1997*), were made in order to increase the extent of induced coagulation and therefore to allow the treatment of larger tumors (*Goldberg et al. 2000*).

The treatment of hepatocellular carcinoma (HCC) in a cirrhotic liver using RF ablation is made easier by the so-called oven effect: the surrounding, densely fibrotic, and poorly vascularized liver tissue and the fibrous capsule hinder thermal conduction away from the target lesion, and thus maintain optimal heat diffusion in the softer, usually well-circumscribed tumoral nodule (*Livraghi et al. 1999*). Conversely, liver metastases are not encapsulated and tend to infiltrate the surrounding well-vascularized liver that can act as a heat sink to limit tissue heating (*Solbiati et al. 1997a*). Therefore RF ablation should aim to necrotize not only the metastatic nodule, but also a 0.5–1.0-cm-thick rim (i.e., a surgical "safety margin") of surrounding liver tissue in order to kill infiltrating tumor undetectable by currently available imaging methods and thus reduce risk of recurrence (*Goldberg et al. 2000*).

6.3
Role of Diagnostic Imaging

Whereas most RF ablation series report a high rate of apparently complete tumor necrosis on initial postablation evaluation, local recurrences probably resulting from a lack of radicality may occur in some cases (*Chopra et al. 2001*). Achieving only partial necrosis implies the need to perform retreatments with increased costs, patient discomfort, greater technical difficulties and higher rates of failure (*DeBaere et al. 2000*).

Diagnostic imaging is of paramount importance in all steps of tumor ablative interventions: (1) detection of lesions and selection of patients for treatment; (2) targeting of lesion(s) with optimal positioning of the energy applicator; (3) immediate assessment of therapeutic result; and (4) long-term follow-up.

In our experience, the use of contrast-enhanced ultrasonography (CEUS) represents a significant improvement in each of these steps and may help to achieve optimal patient management and treatment results.

6.4
Detection of Lesions and Selection of Patients

Early detection and accurate assessment of the extent of neoplastic liver disease at the time of diagnosis or during the course of treatment is crucial for optimal patient management. Given the wide range of treatment options currently available, this may usually result in prolonged survival and a chance for cure. In most centers, patients with previously treated colorectal or other primary cancers may undergo RF ablation of 1-4 metachronous liver metastases, each smaller than 4 cm. Patients with chronic liver disease/cirrhosis may be treated with RF for up to four HCCs and/or dysplastic lesions, in the absence of portal thrombosis and liver function decompensation. Larger HCCs are usually noninvasively treated by means of combined therapies (chemoembolization, ethanol injection, laser, RF).

Cross-sectional imaging modalities such as multiphasic contrast-enhanced helical computed tomography (CT) and dynamic gadolinium-enhanced magnetic resonance imaging (MRI) provide convenient staging of hepatic and extrahepatic neoplastic involvement. Unenhanced B-mode ultrasound (US) represents the most widely available low-cost imaging modality for the screening of liver disease and the guidance of ablation procedures, but is less accurate than CT and MRI in the detection of focal lesions, particularly of smaller ones (less than 1 cm, Figs. 6.1a, 6.2a). With US, poor visualization of lesions may be due to a patient's body habitus, bowel gas distention and inhomogeneity of the liver parenchyma due to cirrhosis or chemotherapy.

Pretreatment CEUS can significantly improve detection and staging of liver tumors. Images and/or movie clips are digitally stored and findings are compared with those of contrast-enhanced axial imaging for maximization of lesion detection and "mapping" of le-

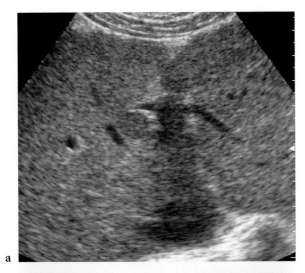

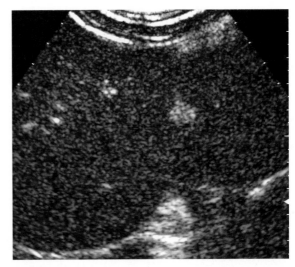

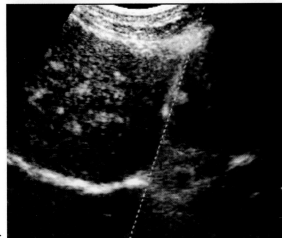

Fig. 6.1 a-c. a A 53-year-old old cirrhotic patient with one 12-mm solid, slightly hypoechoic focal lesion at segment 4, regarded as hepatocellular carcinoma. **b** With CEUS in arterial phase, no focal enhancement is found at segment 4 (suggesting the diagnosis of regenerative nodule for the lesion seen with baseline US), whereas a 9-mm hyperenhancing nodule (invisible with baseline US) is clearly detected at segment 2 and diagnosed as hepatocellular carcinoma. The only way to precisely target this tiny HCC for RF ablation is to repeat CEUS and to guide the cool-tip electrode (Radionics-Tyco, Burlington, MA, USA) into the lesion during the short enhancement time of the arterial phase (**c**)

sions to be targeted during the operating session (Figs. 6.1, 6.2). For patients' pretreatment staging, CEUS can be an extremely valuable tool, particularly for liver metastases. In our experience, increased conspicuity (vs. contrast-enhanced helical CT) for tiny hypovascular metastases was obtained in 12% of patients, with detection of previously invisible lesions in 54% of these cases : this led to a modification in the therapeutic approach since RF was excluded for 38% of these patients.

As a consequence, pretreatment diagnostic work-up should include laboratory tests and tumor markers, conventional and enhanced US and at least one cross-sectional imaging modality (CT and/or MRI) performed no more than 1 week prior to the therapeutic session.

6.5
RF Procedures and Targeting of Lesions

US represents the modality of choice for the guidance of ablative procedures and its benefits include nearly universal availability, portability, ease of use and real-time visualization of electrode placement.

According to our protocol, pretreatment CEUS examination is performed as an initial step of the RF session, during the induction of anesthesia, in order to reproduce mapping of lesions as shown on CT/MRI examinations and to allow real-time lesion targeting. Images and/or movie clips are again digitally stored to be compared with immediate postablation study.

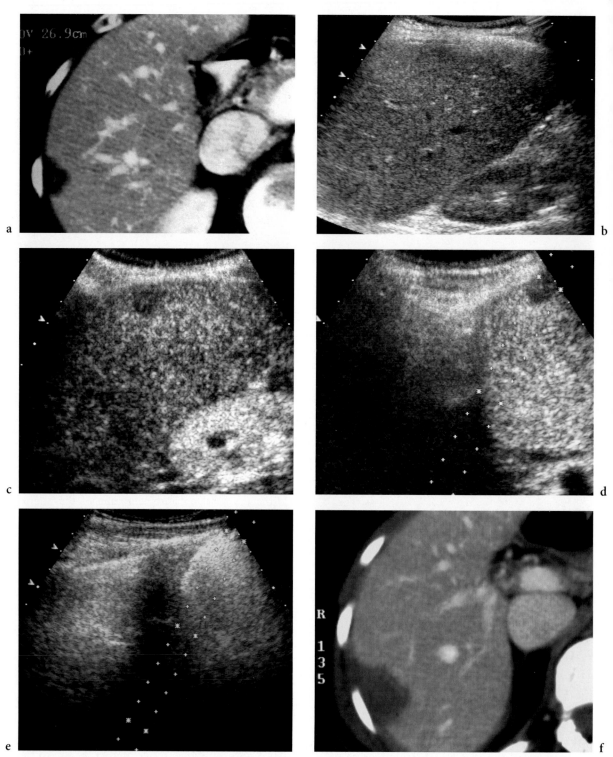

Fig. 6.2 a-f. a In this 49-year-old female patient with history of surgery for breast cancer and multiple cycles of chemotherapy for bone and liver metastases, contrast-enhanced CT shows one residual hypodense 18-mm metastasis at segment 6 in subcapsular location. **b** With unenhanced US the lesion is not clearly identifiable. **c** On CEUS in portal phase a hypoechoic nodule corresponding to the CT finding is clearly detected in subcapsular position. During the same portal phase the target is carried within the *dotted lines* indicating the needle path (**d**) and the RF treatment is performed in 12 min, with abundant gas formation (**e**). Posttreatment CT scan confirms the completeness of ablation, with a hypodense area larger than the original lesion (**f**)

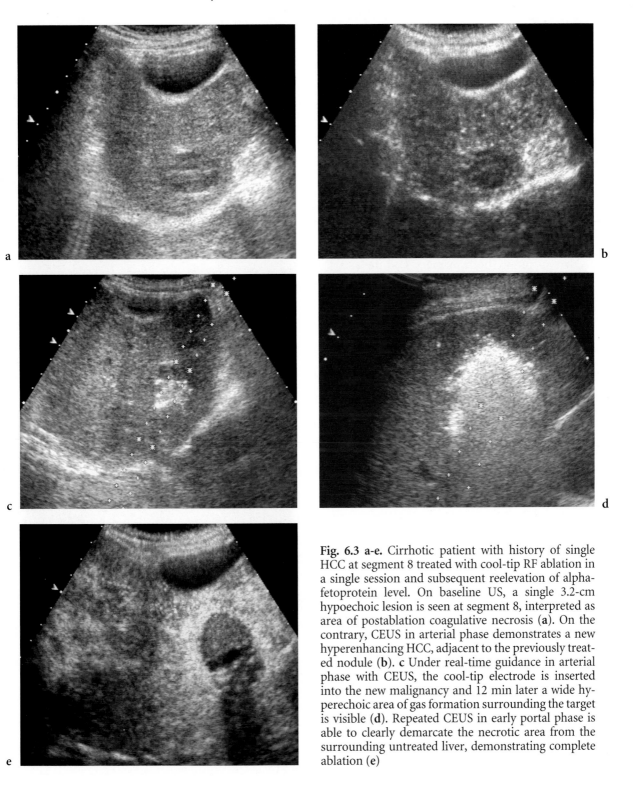

Fig. 6.3 a-e. Cirrhotic patient with history of single HCC at segment 8 treated with cool-tip RF ablation in a single session and subsequent reelevation of alpha-fetoprotein level. On baseline US, a single 3.2-cm hypoechoic lesion is seen at segment 8, interpreted as area of postablation coagulative necrosis (**a**). On the contrary, CEUS in arterial phase demonstrates a new hyperenhancing HCC, adjacent to the previously treated nodule (**b**). **c** Under real-time guidance in arterial phase with CEUS, the cool-tip electrode is inserted into the new malignancy and 12 min later a wide hyperechoic area of gas formation surrounding the target is visible (**d**). Repeated CEUS in early portal phase is able to clearly demarcate the necrotic area from the surrounding untreated liver, demonstrating complete ablation (**e**)

In particularly difficult cases, needle insertion is performed during the specific phase in which the maximum lesion conspicuity is observed : in the arterial phase for hypervascular lesions such as HCCs (Fig. 6.1c) and hypervascular metastases, in the portal or equilibrium phases for hypovascular metastases (Fig. 6.2d). We consider real-time guidance of needle positioning during CEUS mandatory for: (a) small HCCs not visible in cirrhotic liver except as transiently hyperenhancing foci; (b) small subcentimeter metastases barely or not perceptible on unenhanced US but clearly evident as hypoenhancing foci in portal or late phases; (c) areas of residual untreated locally recurrent tumor (both primary and metastatic) in which conventional US cannot allow differentiation between coagulation necrosis and viable tumor (Fig. 6.3).

6.6
Assessment of Therapeutic Response

Sonographic and color/power Doppler findings observed during ablation procedures provide only a gross estimate of the extent of induced coagulation necrosis and therefore are not useful to reliably assess treatment completeness (*Goldberg et al. 2000*). Furthermore, additional repositioning of probes or electrodes may become obscured because during the application of thermal energy a progressively increasing hyperechogenic "cloud" due to gas microbubble formation and tissue vaporization appears around the distal probe and may persist for a few minutes (Fig. 6.4).

The most important imaging finding that suggests complete treatment of a focal liver tumor is the disappearance of any previously visualized vascular enhancement on contrast-enhanced images (*Rhim et al. 2001*). Either biphasic helical CT or dynamic gadolinium-enhanced MRI, although more expensive and less immediate than US, is useful in the assessment of therapeutic efficacy for both hepatoma and metastatic lesions. Good correlation exists between CT and MRI findings, as radiologic–pathologic correlation in experimental and clinical studies demonstrated that

both modalities can predict the extent of coagulation area to within 2–3 mm (*Goldberg et al. 2000*). Being practically unfeasible when ablations are performed in the interventional (either surgical or sonographic) room, contrast-enhanced CT (or less frequently MRI) studies are performed within 1 week following the RF ablation session and compared with baseline examinations to differentiate between ablated

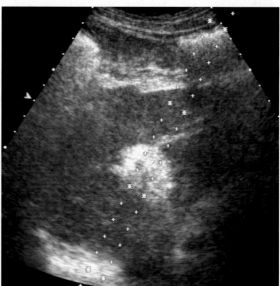

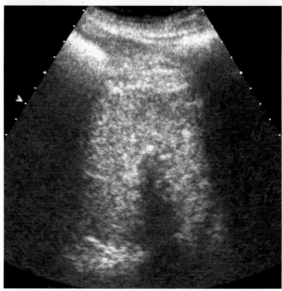

Fig. 6.4 a,b. After ablation, the wide hyperechoic area due to gas formation may lead to overestimation of the actual result of the treatment (**a**). CEUS performed only 5 min after treatment completion can correctly demarcate the real necrotic area from the surrounding liver (**b**)

regions and residual viable tumor requiring additional treatment (*Goldberg et al. 2000*). Coagulation necrosis is displayed on CT as a homogeneously hypoattenuating region, equal in size or larger than the original tumor, with sharp interface with the surrounding parenchyma and lack of neoplastic or parenchymal contrast enhancement in any vascular phase throughout the entire lesion. Hepatic arterial phase images are required for postablation assessment of hypervascular HCCs, whereas differentiation of coagulated areas from hypovascular tumor is usually easier on portal and delayed-phase images. In CT studies performed in the first few days after treatment, a perilesional hyperdense halo is often visible in early-phase images: this finding corresponds on histopathology to an inflammatory reaction to the thermal damage and generally regresses during the first month (*Rhim et al. 2001; Choi et al. 2001*).

On dynamic-enhanced MRI, markedly decreased signal intensity on T2-weighted SE acquisitions is considered the characteristic sign of coagulation necrosis. Necrotic regions with loss of gadolinium enhancement appear as hypointense to the normal enhancing liver. Also with MRI, a uniform peripheral rim of enhancement along the periphery of the treated area does not suggest tumor persistence: unlike CT, this finding may persist for several months. With both contrast-enhanced modalities, partial necrosis manifests generally as nodular or crescentic areas of viable residual neoplastic tissue with the characteristic baseline and enhancement behavior of pretreatment lesions.

CT and MRI assessment of RF ablation of metastases is more difficult than that of hepatoma, due to the hypovascular and infiltrating nature of the tumor. In most cases, confident assessment of complete ablation of a tumor can only be made based upon the necrosis volume exceeding the original lesion and a 0.5–1-cm "safety margin" in every diameter.

Since the introduction of first-generation US contrast agents, color Doppler (CD) and power Doppler (PD) modalities have been used to evaluate the response of hepatocellular carcinoma to interventional treatments, including RF ablation. Initial experiences addressing the usefulness of CE-PD after RF ablation of hepatoma demonstrated the possibility of detecting hypervascular tissue consistent with residual viable tumor with complete specificity and 90% sensitivity (*Choi et al. 2002; Cioni et al. 2001*). Similarly, our group studied patients with liver metastases immediately after ablation and demonstrated that CEUS in CD and PD modes could help differentiate perfused from nonperfused tissue and detect residual tumor, enabling additional treatment sessions in some, but not all cases (*Solbiati et al. 1999*).

More recently, after the introduction of harmonic US, other authors investigated the utility of this technique in combination with first-generation contrast agent after different treatment modalities in patients with hepatoma (*Numata et al. 2001; Ding et al. 2001*). Meloni et al. (2001) demonstrated the superiority of pulse inversion CE-US over CE-PD (sensitivity 23.3% vs 9.3%) in the detection of residual HCC after 4 months of RF ablation. In all these experiences, helical CT was adopted as the "gold standard" and specificity was considered complete (100%) for viable hepatoma when foci of persistent hypervascularity were observed.

Some authors report that when the first RF treatment has not effectively eradicated the tumor, it is extremely difficult to differentiate active tumor from coagulation necrosis and therefore to target residual tumor foci (*DeBaere et al. 2000*).

In our protocol, immediate postablation evaluation using CEUS is performed 5–10 min after the assumed completion of the RF session, with the patient still under general anesthesia. As depicted on contrast-enhanced CT and MRI, a thin and uniform enhancing rim is usually visible along the periphery of the necrotic area, which should not be mistaken for tumor. Comparison of immediate postablation images with stored preablation scans is mandatory. Residual viable hepatoma is suspected when a portion of the original lesion maintains hypervascularity in the arterial phase (Figs. 6.5, 6.6). As with helical CT, residual untreated metastatic lesions sometimes appear indistinguishable from necrosis in the portal and equilibrium phases : on CEUS, evaluation of the early phase is important since vi-

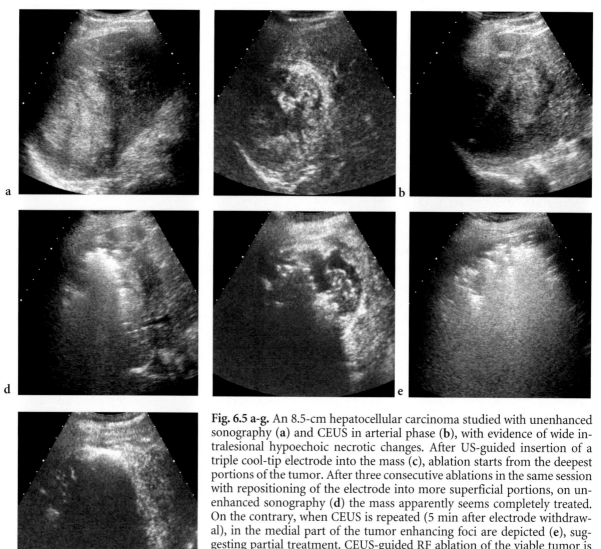

Fig. 6.5 a-g. An 8.5-cm hepatocellular carcinoma studied with unenhanced sonography (**a**) and CEUS in arterial phase (**b**), with evidence of wide intralesional hypoechoic necrotic changes. After US-guided insertion of a triple cool-tip electrode into the mass (**c**), ablation starts from the deepest portions of the tumor. After three consecutive ablations in the same session with repositioning of the electrode into more superficial portions, on unenhanced sonography (**d**) the mass apparently seems completely treated. On the contrary, when CEUS is repeated (5 min after electrode withdrawal), in the medial part of the tumor enhancing foci are depicted (**e**), suggesting partial treatment. CEUS-guided RF ablation of the viable tumor is performed in the same session with a huge hyperechoic area due to gas formation visible with unenhanced US (**f**). CEUS repeated once more demarcates the real necrotic area which has the same size of the original mass ("oven effect") demonstrating complete ablation (**g**)

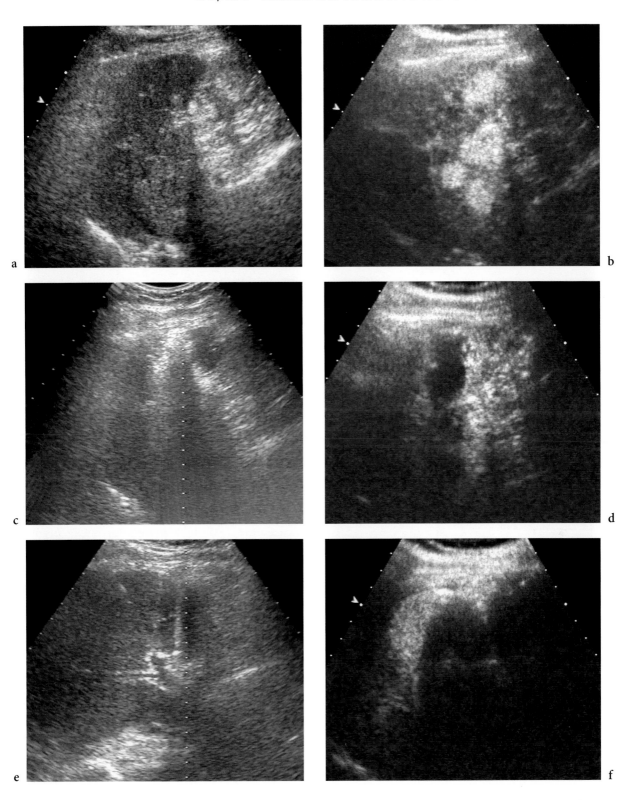

Fig. 6.6 a-f. A 75-year-old cirrhotic patient with multifocal HCC. **a** On unenhanced sonography, no mass is clearly demonstrated. **b** CEUS shows many tiny hyperenhancing foci in arterial phase grouped in segments 4 and 7. RF ablation is performed (**c**) and, at the end of the treatment, CEUS is repeated (**d**) showing some residual foci of untreated HCC. Under CEUS-guidance, further RF ablation is performed in the same session and posttreatment CEUS finally shows complete result (**e, f**)

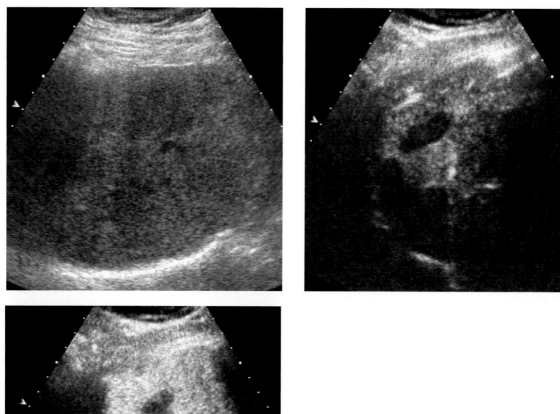

Fig. 6.7 a-c. Sonographic study of a patient treated 30 days previously for large colorectal metastasis at segment 8. Baseline US is unable to differentiate treated from untreated areas (**a**). **b** CEUS in arterial phase shows a triangular enhancing area between two unenhancing areas which disappears (becoming hypoechoic) in portal phase (**c**). This is a clear-cut demonstration of residual viable metastatic tissue between posttreatment necrotic areas

able tumor shows weak but perceptible enhancement (Fig. 6.7). If even questionable residual tumor foci with enhancement or vascular supply are depicted, immediate CEUS-guided targeted retreatment is carried out. Treatment is stopped only when complete avascularity is demonstrated.

Over an 18-month study period in our institution, in 176 of 199 liver malignancies treated, no residual tumor was found on CEUS: of these, CT depicted residual foci only in 4 cases, all of which were very small (0.8–1.7 cm). On the other hand, in the remaining 23 tumors, single or multiple (1.0–2.2 cm) residual foci were detected and immediately submitted to

additional RF application in the same session until no further residual enhancement was detectable: in 2 cases (8.7%) a 1.2–1.9-cm residual tumor was depicted at CT. With the routine adoption of CEUS as the only technical improvement, our final most impressive result is a 5.1% rate (6/119 lesions) of partial necrosis, in comparison with a 16.1% rate achieved from 1994 to August 2000 (prior to the introduction of CEUS for the real-time management of ablations) for 429 hepatocellular and metastatic lesions. This approach greatly simplifies patient management and reduces costs by decreasing both the number of RF procedures and follow-up examinations.

References

Buscarini L, Buscarini E, Di Stasi M, Vallisa D, Quaretti P, Rocca A (2001) Percutaneous radiofrequency ablation of small hepatocellular carcinoma: long-term results. Eur Radiol 11: 914-92

Choi H, Loyer EM, DuBrow RA, et al (2001) Radio-frequency ablation of liver tumors: assessment of therapeutic response and complications. Radiographics 21: S41-S54

Choi D, Lim HK, Kim SH, et al (2000) Hepatocellular carcinoma treated with percutaneous radio-frequency ablation: usefulness of power Doppler US with a microbubble contrast agent in evaluation of therapeutic response-preliminary study. Radiology 217:558-563

Chopra S, Dodd GD 3rd, Chintapalli KN, Leyendecker JR, Karahan OI, Rhim H (2001) Tumor recurrence after radiofrequency thermal ablation of hepatic tumors: spectrum of findings on dual-phase contrast-enhanced CT. AJR 177:381-387

Cioni D, Lencioni R, Rossi S, Garbagnati F, Donati F, Crocetti L, Bartolozzi C (2001) Radiofrequency thermal ablation of hepatocellular carcinoma: using contrast-enhanced harmonic power Doppler sonography to assess treatment outcome. AJR 177:783-788

De Baere T, Elias D, Dromain C, et al (2000) Radiofrequency ablation of 100 hepatic metastases with a mean follow-up of more than 1 year. AJR 175:1619-1625

Ding H, Kudo M, Onda H, et al (2001) Evaluation of posttreatment response of hepatocellular carcinoma with contrast-enhanced coded phase-inversion harmonic US. Comparison with dynamic CT. Radiology 221:712-730

Dodd GD 3rd, Soulen MC, Kane RA, et al (2000) Minimally invasive treatment of malignant hepatic tumors: at the threshold of a major breakthrough. Radiographics 20:9-27

Goldberg SN, Gazelle GS, Solbiati L, Rittman WJ, Mueller PR (1996) Radiofrequency tissue ablation: increased lesion diameter with a perfusion electrode. Acad Radiol 3:636-644

Goldberg SN, Solbiati L, Hahn PF, Cosman E, Conrad JE, Fogle R, Gazelle GS (1998) Large-volume tissue ablation with radiofrequency by using a clustered, internally cooled electrode technique: laboratory and clinical experience in liver metastases. Radiology 209:371-379

Goldberg SN, Stein MC, Gazelle GS, Sheiman RG, Kruskal JB, Clouse ME (1999) Percutaneous radiofrequency tissue ablation: optimization of pulsed-radiofrequency technique to increase coagulation necrosis. J Vasc Interv Radiol 10:907-916

Goldberg SN, Gazelle GS, Compton CC, Mueller PR, Tanabe KK (2000) Treatment of intrahepatic malignancy with radiofrequency ablation: radiologic-pathologic correlation. Cancer 88:2452-2463

Livraghi T, Goldberg SN, Monti F, et al (1997) Saline-enhanced radio-frequency tissue ablation in the treatment of liver metastases. Radiology 202:205-210

Livraghi T, Goldberg SN, Lazzaroni S, Meloni F, Solbiati L, Gazelle GS (1999) Small hepatocellular carcinoma: treatment with radiofrequency ablation versus ethanol injection. Radiology 210:655-661

Livraghi T, Goldberg SN, Lazzaroni S, Meloni F, Ierace T, Solbiati L, Gazelle GS (2000) Hepatocellular carcinoma: radiofrequency ablation of medium and large lesions. Radiology 214:761-768

Livraghi T, Goldberg SN, Solbiati L, Meloni F, Ierace T, Gazelle GS (2001) Percutaneous radio-frequency ablation of liver metastases from breast cancer: initial experience in 24 patients. Radiology 220:145-149

Meloni MF, Goldberg SN, Livraghi T, et al (2001) Hepatocellular carcinoma treated with radiofrequency ablation. Comparision of pulse inversion contrast-enhanced harmonic sonography, contrast-enhanced power Doppler sonography and helical CT. AJR 177:375-380

Numata K, Tanaka K, Kiba T, et al (2001) Using contrast-enhanced sonography to assess the effectiveness of transcatheter arterial embolization for hepatocellular carcinoma. AJR 176:1199-1205

Rhim H, Goldberg SN, Dodd Gd 3rd, Solbiati L, Lim HK, Tonolini M, Cho OK (2001) Essential techniques for successful radiofrequency thermal ablation of malignant hepatic tumors. Radiographics 21: S17-31

Solbiati L, Goldberg SN, Ierace T, et al (1997a) Hepatic metastases : percutaneous radio-frequency ablation with cooled-tip electrodes. Radiology 205:367-373

Solbiati L, Ierace T, Goldberg SN, et al (1997b) Percutaneous US-guided radio-frequency tissue ablation of liver metastases: Treatment and follow-up in 16 patients. Radiology 202:195-203

Solbiati L, Goldberg SN, Ierace T, Della Noce M, Livraghi T, Gazelle GS (1999) Radio-frequency ablation of hepatic metastases: postprocedural assessment with a US microbubble contrast agent – early experience. Radiology 211:643-649

Solbiati L, Livraghi T, Goldberg SN, et al (2001) Percutaneous radio-frequency ablation of hepatic metastases from colorectal cancer: long-term results in 117 patients. Radiology 221:159-166

Solbiati L, Tonolini M, Cova L, Goldberg SN (2001) The role of contrast-enhanced ultrasound in the detection of focal liver lesions. Eur Radiol 11[Suppl 3]: E15-E26

7   Hands-on Contrast Ultrasound

J.M. Correas, O. Hélénon

Liver contrast-enhanced ultrasonography (CEUS) is leaving the stage of a "rescue" examination in cases of technical failure to become a full imaging modality, like computed tomography (CT) and magnetic resonance imaging (MRI). The success of this new modality requires that some guidelines are followed so that the rate of failure or misdiagnosis is reduced.

7.1
Tips and Tricks

7.1.1
Organization of Contrast-Enhanced US

Liver CEUS requires some reorganization in a conventional US department, because it is slightly longer than a routine US examination (about 30 min) and necessitates the insertion of an intravenous (IV) catheter. CEUS can be scheduled at the end of US sessions, but in most institutions, the US sessions are fully booked in advance. In our department, one to two morning US sessions per week are dedicated to CEUS, with the participation of a trained technologist or nurse to prepare and administer the US contrast agent (USCA). Most of the requests for liver CEUS are made by hepatologists and oncologists, aware of the potentials of this new imaging modality. All patients sign an informed consent form and can discuss the procedure with either the technologist or the radiologist. In our experience, no patient has refused the insertion of an IV catheter.

7.1.2.
Intravenous Access

The IV line requires some precautions: the size of the catheter should be at least 20 Gauges, the site of puncture should be as close as possible to the elbow. The length of the extension tubing should be shortened as much as possible. A three-way stopcock can be directly inserted on the IV catheter with a 10-ml saline syringe on the side port. The permeability of the IV line must be checked before the administration of the USCA using a bolus injection of saline.

7.1.3
Preparation of the USCA

Most USCAs are made with microbubbles. Unlike iodinated contrast agents or MRI contrast agents, these microbubbles are very fragile and can be destroyed by any pressure excess. Therefore, the vial must be ventilated during reconstitution to avoid excessive internal pressure. USCA efficacy is also reduced if excessive pressure is applied by the plunger during bolus administration, for example, when the IV line is partially occluded. Any manipulation of the compound after reconstitution (such as dilution or reinjection in a different vial or syringe) will alter the microbubble stability. While withdrawn into the syringe, rapid administration of the compoundis recommended.

7.1.4
The USCAs

Two USCAs are currently approved for liver CEUS; Levovist® (Schering SA, Germany) and SonoVue® (Bracco, Italy). Levovist® was approved a few years ago and is available in most western European countries, Japan and Canada. It is based on air microbubbles stabilized with a galactose matrix and palmitic acid. SonoVue® has been approved recently and has become available in many European countries. The microbubbles are filled with a perfluorocarbon gas, sulfur hexafluoride, and stabilized with various surfactants and palmitic acid. There is no comparative study published as yet. The choice of USCA depends on some specific contra-indications and indications as well as on the availability of the compound. Both of these USCAs should not be administered in children younger than 15 years as well as in pregnant or lactating women, as a general precaution. Otherwise, USCAs are very well tolerated.

Levovist® is contraindicated in cases of galactosemia, which is a very rare recessive autosomal disease due to a deficit in galactose-1-phosphate-uridyl-transferase. Two doses are available (2.5- and 4-g vials) that can be reconstituted at different concentrations of 200, 300 and 400 mg/ml by adding variable volumes of sterile water through a MiniSpike®. Levovist® should be administered within 2 min of reconstitution, since the microbubble population changes fast. The 300 mg/ml concentration can be used for both Doppler and nonlinear imaging, while the 400 mg/ml concentration is more appropriate for nonlinear imaging. For Doppler indications, the 2.5-g vial is appropriate and the injection rate must be adapted to the level of Doppler signal enhancement. Short boluses of 0.5–1 ml can be repeated. If an electric pump syringe is available, Levovist® can be injected with a small bolus of 1 ml followed by an infusion of 1 ml/min. The flow rate must be adapted to the contrast enhancement.

For nonlinear applications, the 2.5-g vial may be used in thin patients while the 4-g vial is preferred in large patients and in cases of obesity or cirrhosis, to provide the best and most reliable enhancement possible. The 300 mg/ml or the 400 mg/ml concentration can be used, with a preference for 400 mg/ml in difficult cases in our experience.

SonoVue® is contraindicated in cases of right-to-left shunts, severe increase in pulmonary artery blood pressure, uncontrolled hypertension and adult respiratory distress syndrome. Special care should be taken in cases of stress-enhanced echocardiography, severe cardiac diseases including severe heart failure and severe lung diseases.

SonoVue® is reconstituted by injecting 5 ml saline through a MiniSpike®. Within the vial, the compound is stable for a few hours (< 6 h). For Doppler indications, it can be administered using short boluses of 0.6–1 ml , but the best results are obtained using slow infusions at a rate of 0.5–1 ml/min, depending on the signal enhancement. For nonlinear imaging, bolus injections provide a stronger enhancement. The recommended dose of 2.4 ml can be repeated twice. It can be reduced to 1–1.5 ml to allow multiple bolus studies and complete liver scanning during arterial phase.

7.1.5
Scanning Techniques and Settings

Conventional color and Doppler US are facing a major limitation due to blooming artifacts. These artifacts can be reduced using a slower USCA injection rate and a combination of changes in the Doppler settings. This combination can include a slight reduction of the acoustic power (reflected by the mechanical index), an increase in the Doppler filters and the pulse repetition frequency, a decrease in the Doppler gains and in the color persistence, and an increase in the line density.

Nonlinear imaging settings were optimized depending on the microbubble acoustic properties. A large difference is observed between the two USCAs: with the Levovist®, a strong nonlinear response is obtained only at high acoustic power, resulting in destruction of most of the microbubbles within the US field. The position of the focal zone is critical, and is usually located at 2/3 of the liver depth. The microbubbles can be found up to 20 min after injection in the absence of destruction, due to some specific adherence to the liver sinusoids.

The technique of scanning becomes critical because the renewal of the microbubble population is limited. The liver must be scanned using sweeps covering the entire organ with a gentle displacement of the probe toward the same direction. It is not possible to move back to an area previously imaged in the same sweep because no enhancement will be observed. It is necessary to define the placement of the transducer before the injection for each sweep, and eventually to mark the start and end of each on the patient skin. It is useful to train the patient to take reproducible deep in-breaths to avoid starting the scan in the middle of the liver. Alternative scans on the right and left liver lobes allow reperfusion of the liver parenchyma and an increase in the number of sweeps (Fig. 7.1). The imaging technique should be adapted to the clinical indication with two different situations: detection of lesions or characterization of a known liver mass.

7.1.6
Liver CEUS using Levovist®

7.1.6.1
Detection of Liver Masses using Levovist®

Detection is best performed scanning the liver during the late phase, i.e., starting approximately 2 min after the administration of the USCA. The examination is performed at high mechanical index (MI >1) using alternate right and left sweeps, covering the entire liver. The position of the focal zone is usually at two-thirds of the liver depth. However, in case of suspicion of a superficial lesion, the focal zone can be set at the one-third of the liver depth at the beginning of the examination, and moved down for later sweeps. Each sweep should be carefully reviewed using the cineloop, as there is no rush to go to the next sweep. The sweep can be stored on the internal hard disk or on the network for further study.

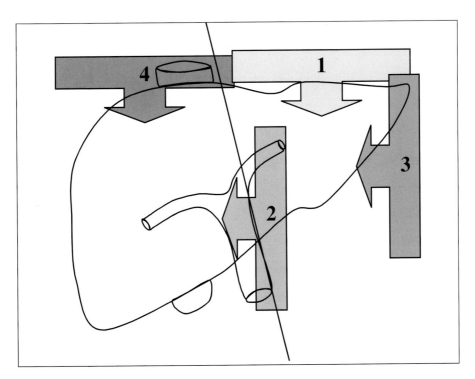

Fig. 7.1. During late-phase imaging with Levovist®, a precise scanning technique improves the number of sweeps. Alternative scans on the right and left liver allow reperfusion of the liver parenchyma. After each acquisition, the entire cineloop should be carefully reviewed. The delay between each sweep is about 20–30 s. The following sequence can be proposed: first sweep, oblique transverse scanon the left liver (top to bottom direction); second sweep, sagittal sweep on the right liver (left to right direction), starting at the level of the portal vein; third sweep, sagittal sweep on the left liver (left to right direction); fourth sweep, oblique transverse scan on the right liver (top to bottom direction)

7.1.6.2
Characterization of a Known Liver Mass Using Levovist®

It is possible to scan the lesion during the arterial phase, lowering the pulse repetition frequency (e.g., 5 frames per second) and reducing the mechanical index to 0.7–0.8, depending on the location of the lesion. The highest dose and concentration are recommended. The focal zone is then located immediately beyond the lesion. A late-phase scan is still possible starting on the other lobe for the detection of additional masses, with the highest mechanical index available. The area of the studied mass should be scanned later to allow fresh microbubbles to refill the hepatic sinusoids.

7.1.7
Liver CEUS using SonoVue®

On the contrary, SonoVue® provides a nonlinear response at low acoustic power. Starting with almost no signal from the tissue, the arrival of the compound is visualized with real-time imaging and allows multiple scanning in different planes. This technique is much easier to perform when apnea is not reproducible, or when the position of the suspected lesion is unknown. However, it is difficult to achieve accurate assessment of the deep parenchyma along with an appropriate preservation despite high gain settings. Moreover, it is not possible to achieve late-phase imaging with SonoVue®, because there is no or little pooling of the microbubbles in the liver sinusoids. The location of the focal zone is less critical, and usually settled at two-thirds of the liver depth.

7.1.7.1
Detection of Liver Masses Using SonoVue®

The best phase to achieve detection of liver masses is during portal phase, starting approximately 2–3 min after the injection of the US-CA. The examination is performed at low mechanical index (MI 0.1–0.2). Alternate right and left sweeps are not necessary as the destruction is limited. The focal zone can be moved up and down depending on the areas of suspicion. The sweeps should be carefully reviewed using the cineloop, and stored for further analysis. A major difficulty is caused by poor signal intensity obtained from the deep liver. After scanning the two-third anterior parenchyma, the mechanical index can be increased to 0.2–0.3.

7.1.7.2
Characterization of a Known Liver Mass Using SonoVue®

The lesion is easily studied during all enhancement phases (and particularly during arterial phase) because of the real-time imaging and the multiple sweeps available (Fig. 7.2). The pulse repetition frequency can be maintained as high as possible and the mechanical index is reduced to 0.1–0.2. It can be increased slightly when the contrast effect disappears. The focal zone is located beyond the lesion. The final diagnosis relies on arterial phase enhancement and appearance during the portal phase.

7.2
Limitations

The major limitations of CEUS of the liver are due to anatomical factors and microbubble fragility. Parenchyma that cannot be easily reached by the US pulse remains difficult to assess despite the injection of a USCA. Such a limitation occurs for subdiaphragmatic segments because of interposition of the pleura and the lungs, and in enlarged attenuating liver. At high mechanical index, the resonance of Levovist® microbubbles is difficult to achieve due to attenuation of the acoustic pressure. Simultaneously, the nonlinear acoustic response from the solid tissue increases masking the signals from the microbubbles. At low mechanical index, the nonlinear response from the deep liver tissue can be neglected. However, the signal obtained from the microbubbles is extremely low due to attenuation phenomena. The presence of microbubbles at the level of the liver assumes correct storage of the compound, adequate preparation and administra-

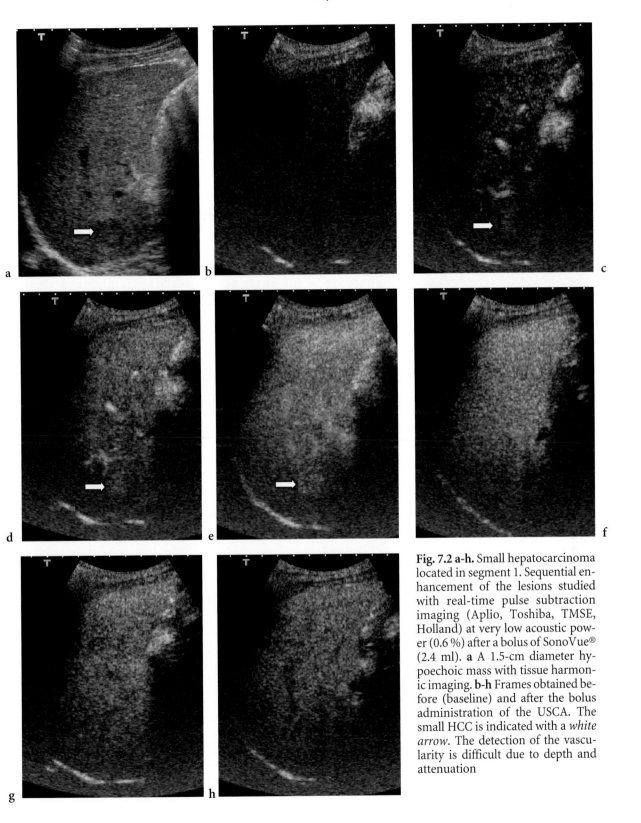

Fig. 7.2 a-h. Small hepatocarcinoma located in segment 1. Sequential enhancement of the lesions studied with real-time pulse subtraction imaging (Aplio, Toshiba, TMSE, Holland) at very low acoustic power (0.6 %) after a bolus of SonoVue® (2.4 ml). **a** A 1.5-cm diameter hypoechoic mass with tissue harmonic imaging. **b-h** Frames obtained before (baseline) and after the bolus administration of the USCA. The small HCC is indicated with a *white arrow*. The detection of the vascularity is difficult due to depth and attenuation

tion of the microbubbles. A partially occluded peripheral vein, low cardiac output, and large extension tubing reduce largely the contrast enhancement in the large vessels and in the parenchyma.

7.3
Artifacts and Pitfalls

The performance of liver CEUS relies on two critical factors: the intensity and the homogeneity of the enhancement provided by the USCA. Pitfalls can result from any alteration of these two factors. The intensity of the enhancement depends on the acoustic properties and pharmacokinetics of the microbubbles. The mechanical index plays a key role, as the nonlinear response from the USCA increases with the local acoustic power until the stage of microbubble disruption. The homogeneity of the enhancement depends on the distribution of the microbubbles and the uniformity of the acoustic energy within the imaging plane. The position of the focal zone is usually the area where the maximum enhancement is detected. In large venous structures, homogeneity also varies with the distribution of the microbubbles within the lumen and with the blood flow pattern.

At high mechanical index (MI >0.5), the main artifacts and pitfalls are:

- Microbubble destruction due to previous scans or slow-moving probe
- Attenuation of the enhancement with depth
- Heterogeneity of the enhancement: insufficient superficial subcapsular enhancement, hypoenhancing areas with sharp borders that can mimic pseudonodules
- Heterogeneous enhancement in venous structures.

At low mechanical index (MI <0.5), the main artifacts and pitfalls are:
- Low enhancement intensity
- Attenuation of the enhancement with depth.

Lesions can also exhibit an atypical enhancement pattern with both imaging techniques.

7.3.1
Heterogeneous Enhancement

Heterogeneous enhancement is mainly seen with high mechanical index nonlinear imaging, such as pulse inversion imaging.

7.3.1.1
Destruction of the Microbubbles

The alternate low and high enhancement is due to slow transducer displacement, with the two frames acquired on the same parenchyma. The first frame exhibits a strong enhancement because of the microbubble destruction and the following one is back to baseline, due to the almost complete destruction of the agent on the first frame (Fig. 7.3). When two sweeps are rapidly performed with different angles on the same area during late-phase Levovist® imaging, the territory where microbubbles were previously destroyed appears as a dark weakly enhancing area with sharp edges (Fig. 7.4). Artifacts due to microbubble destruction are more homogeneous with liver-specific USCAs (such as NC 100100, Sonazoid®, Amersham; Fig. 7.5).

7.3.1.2
Effect of Attenuation and Focal Zone Position

The attenuation of the US beam results from the combination of liver intrinsic acoustic properties (steatosis, fibrosis and increased depth), the concentration and acoustic properties of the microbubbles and the level of the acoustic power. The deeper parenchyma exhibits little enhancement (Fig. 7.6). The position of the focal zone and the mechanical index can be varied to increase the visibility of the deep segments. When the attenuation is due to the excess of microbubbles, a second sweep on the same area might solve the limited penetration of the US beam by destroying superficial USCA. The limited assessment of deep liver parenchyma is even increasing a low mechanical index. With a mechanical index lower than 0.2, the visibility of small lesions at more than 14 cm depth is almost impossible with nonlinear imaging (Fig. 7.2). New imaging techniques such as Agent Detection Imaging® provide a more uniform field of enhancement.

Typically, the superficial subcapsular parenchyma and the deep areas exhibit little contrast while the midparenchyma at the level of the focal zone is strongly enhanced (Fig. 7.6). During late-phase Levovist® imaging, hypo-enhanced areas with sharp edges indicate previous sweeps performed with a different orientation of the transducer.

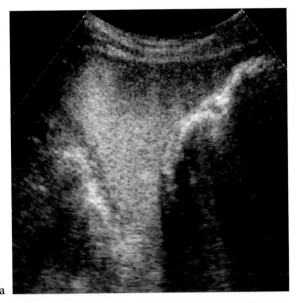
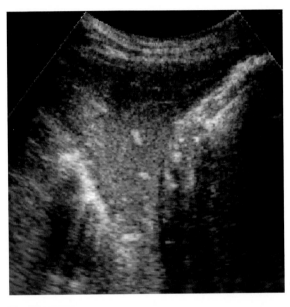

Fig. 7.3 a,b. Variability of the enhancement observed on two consecutive frames (sagittal view on the left liver) observed using pulse inversion imaging at high mechanical index (1.4) following Levovist® injection (4 g, 400 mg/ml). The first frame (**a**) exhibits a strong enhancement due to microbubble resonance and destruction. The consecutive frame (**b**) is obtained after little displacement of the probe. There is almost no enhancement due to previous destruction of the microbubbles in the imaging plane

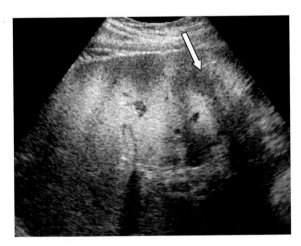
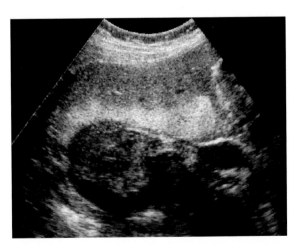

Fig. 7.4. Heterogeneous enhancement due to previous destruction of the microbubble (pulse inversion imaging, high MI, Levovist® 4 g, 400 mg/ml). Sharp linear defect territory (*white arrow*) owing to prior orthogonal acquisition with microbubble destruction

Fig. 7.5. Destruction of microbubbles at high MI (0.8) following the administration of a liver-specific USCA (NC 100100, Sonazoid®, Amersham). The propagation of the destructive front wave on the previous scan produces a more homogeneous destruction on the superficial parenchyma, with preservation of the contrast agent in the deep portions of the liver

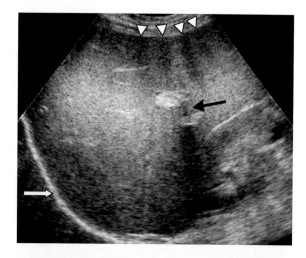

Fig. 7.6. Heterogeneous enhancement (right transverse view, pulse inversion imaging, high MI, Levovist® 4 g, 400 mg/ml). This frame combines several artifacts: poor enhancement on the deep parenchyma (*white arrow*), heterogeneous subcutaneous enhancement due to inhomogeneity of the acoustic energy and focal zone position (*white arrowhead*), and shadowing artifact due to liver sinus interposition (*black arrow*)

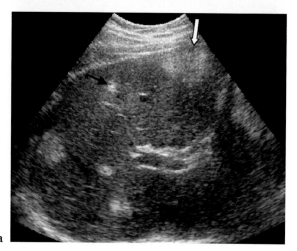

a

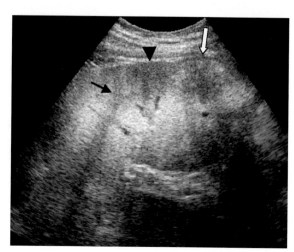

b

Fig. 7.7 a,b. Hyperechoic metastases from a colon carcinoma. **a** B-mode transverse view on the right liver, with 3 hyperechoic masses and a calcification (*black arrow*). **b** Same view obtained during late phase imaging (pulse inversion imaging, high MI, Levovist® 4 g, 400 mg/ml). The metastases are slightly hypoechoic due to the enhancement of the normal liver (*white arrow* on the superficial mass). However, an adjacent round defect is detected on the subcapsular area (*arrowhead*) on the postcontrast study. This lesion was not seen on CT and MRI and corresponds to a pseudolesion with ill-defined borders, due to the heterogeneous subcapsular enhancement. The hyperechoic deeper lesion is no longer visible. Note the increased visibility of the shadowing due to the small calcification (*black arrow*)

7.3.1.3
Pseudomasses

Sometimes, the combination of a heterogeneous deposition of the USCA and the alteration of the US beam uniformity due to subcutaneous fat can mimic the presence of lesions (Figs. 7.4, 7.6, 7.7). Such pseudomasses are ill-defined and not found on multiple sweeps performed with other angles of view. This effect is minimized at low mechanical index.

7.3.1.4
Atypical Enhancement Pattern

Many lesions with different histopathology can exhibit the same enhancement pattern. Hypervascular enhancement can be found during arterial phase in hypervascular metastases in cancer patients, in hepatocellular carcinomas in patients with cirrhosis or in focal nodular hyperplasia in women with no history of disease. However, this pattern is not specific of

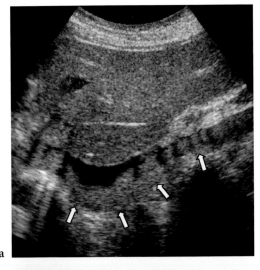
a

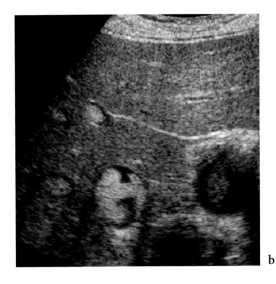
b

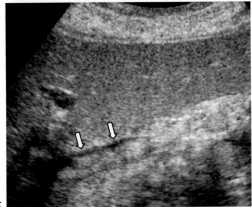
c

Fig. 7.8 a-c. Heterogeneous venous enhancement, following Levovist® injection (pulse inversion imaging, high MI). **a,b** Longitudinal view of the inferior vena cava. The microbubbles follow the blood flow and are pushed down by the ultrasound beam (*white arrows*). **c** Longitudinal view of the portal vein. The vessel lumen is not completely filled by the contrast agent (anterior wall, *white arrows*), but there is no partial thrombosis

malignancy and was also observed in our experience in cases of hypervascular hemangiomas, in regenerative nodular hyperplasia or in dysplastic nodules. Hepatocellular carcinomas can also be found in patients without cirrhosis.

Most malignant hypervascular lesions should appear as hypoechoic compared to the normally enhanced surrounding liver on late-phase imaging. USCA with little or no late-phase imaging will not detect the hypoechogenicity of malignant lesions during the late phase. Hyperechoic masses, such as metastases, can be missed during late-phase scanning due to the enhancement of the normal surrounding liver. The increased backscatter of the normal liver tissue will match the poorly enhancing hyperechoic mass (Fig. 7.7). Therefore baseline scanning with the best available technology is mandatory.

7.3.1.5
Enhancement of Large Veins

Heterogeneous enhancement of the large venous structures is usual using a high-mechanical index imaging modality. The blood flow and distribution of the microbubbles within the vessel lumen, combined with heterogeneous destruction, can create enhancement defects (Fig. 7.8). However, the contrast-enhanced lumen varies with time and scanning planes. The detection of complete or partial thrombosis is best achieved in most cases using conventional gray-scale imaging such as nonlinear imaging modalities alone or combined with compounding techniques.

In conclusion, liver CEUS is a new imaging modality that requires specific training for the best possible results to be achieved. Some simple tips and tricks can really improve the level of contrast enhancement. Artifacts and pitfalls should be known so as to avoid misdiagnosis.